AF729306

INTERNET OF THINGS AND MACHINE LEARNING

INTELLIGENT INFORMATION RETRIEVAL FOR HEALTHCARE SYSTEMS

INTERNET OF THINGS AND MACHINE LEARNING

Additional books and e-books in this series can be found on Nova's website under the Series tab.

INTERNET OF THINGS AND MACHINE LEARNING

INTELLIGENT INFORMATION RETRIEVAL FOR HEALTHCARE SYSTEMS

PARMA NAND

ARUN PRAKASH AGRAWAL

ANKUR CHOUDHARY

AND

VISHAL JAIN

EDITORS

nova science publishers
New York

Copyright © 2021 by Nova Science Publishers, Inc.
DOI: https://doi.org/10.52305/ULIQ1795

All rights reserved. No part of this book may be reproduced, stored in a retrieval system or transmitted in any form or by any means: electronic, electrostatic, magnetic, tape, mechanical photocopying, recording or otherwise without the written permission of the Publisher.

We have partnered with Copyright Clearance Center to make it easy for you to obtain permissions to reuse content from this publication. Simply navigate to this publication's page on Nova's website and locate the "Get Permission" button below the title description. This button is linked directly to the title's permission page on copyright.com. Alternatively, you can visit copyright.com and search by title, ISBN, or ISSN.

For further questions about using the service on copyright.com, please contact:
Copyright Clearance Center
Phone: +1-(978) 750-8400 Fax: +1-(978) 750-4470 E-mail: info@copyright.com.

NOTICE TO THE READER

The Publisher has taken reasonable care in the preparation of this book, but makes no expressed or implied warranty of any kind and assumes no responsibility for any errors or omissions. No liability is assumed for incidental or consequential damages in connection with or arising out of information contained in this book. The Publisher shall not be liable for any special, consequential, or exemplary damages resulting, in whole or in part, from the readers' use of, or reliance upon, this material. Any parts of this book based on government reports are so indicated and copyright is claimed for those parts to the extent applicable to compilations of such works.

Independent verification should be sought for any data, advice or recommendations contained in this book. In addition, no responsibility is assumed by the Publisher for any injury and/or damage to persons or property arising from any methods, products, instructions, ideas or otherwise contained in this publication.

This publication is designed to provide accurate and authoritative information with regard to the subject matter covered herein. It is sold with the clear understanding that the Publisher is not engaged in rendering legal or any other professional services. If legal or any other expert assistance is required, the services of a competent person should be sought. FROM A DECLARATION OF PARTICIPANTS JOINTLY ADOPTED BY A COMMITTEE OF THE AMERICAN BAR ASSOCIATION AND A COMMITTEE OF PUBLISHERS.

Additional color graphics may be available in the e-book version of this book.

Library of Congress Cataloging-in-Publication Data

ISBN: 978-1-68507-301-5

Published by Nova Science Publishers, Inc. † New York

CONTENTS

PREFACE

Ontology–based information extraction is considered as an effective method to improve the performance of information extraction (IE) systems. For research and disbursal of customized healthcare services, a major challenge is to efficiently retrieve and analyze the individual patient data from a large volume of heterogeneous data over a long span of time. This requires effective ontology-based information retrieval approaches for clinical information systems. This book is an attempt to highlight the key advances in ontology-based information retrieval techniques especially in the healthcare domain. The varied chapters attempt to uncover the current challenges in the application of ontology-based information retrieval techniques to the healthcare systems. The book shall be first of its kind that highlights only the ontology driven information retrieval mechanisms and techniques being applied to healthcare as well as clinical information systems. The book can serve as a potential textbook for courses in healthcare systems. It can also serve as a reference book to medical practitioners as well as researchers involved in implementing as well as providing customized health care solutions to patients.

In Chapter 1, the architecture of an information retrieval system for small healthcare centers and clinics is proposed. The system consists of sensors to collect data, an encrypted blockchain cloud gives security and data privacy to create links and transmit data between sensors, and analytical tools are to process, retrieve and evaluate the health condition of the patient. Chapter 2 gives on overview for systematic allotment of zones to the districts and automated policy formulation for the districts by using ontological inference done through the Drool's reasoner. In the Chapter 3, service computing, the necessity for service computing, capabilities and applications of carrier computing, security and privateness issues, and Trust associated problems in fitness care services are certainly represented. Chapter 4 depicts the literature survey of various DL models, different CA methods, the standard methods of predicting these diseases, and provides the need to select this classifier to address this problem. Chapter 5 discusses the novel approach of Health Monitoring System. In the Chapter 6 authors have discussed different architectures and quality requirements that are essential for IoT applications. Authors have illustrated and included three of the best use cases of the healthcare field and discussed its quality requirements. Chapter 7 discusses the various aspects of data privacy and security in Healthcare. Chapter 8 this chapter deals with the scientific analysis of Yajna and Mantra and it has been recorded that almost an all the important chemical elements required for human health are present in Yajna ashes. Chapter 9 mainly focuses on major points in the development of automatic speech and text recognition. Proposed text conversion is also a factor used in speech recognition from last few years. Chapter 10 discusses about the storing and maintaining the smart healthcare in IoT environment.

In: Intelligent Information Retrieval ... ISBN: 978-1-68507-301-5
Editors: Parma Nand et al. © 2021 Nova Science Publishers, Inc.

Chapter 1

Ontology-Based Information Retrieval System Using Blockchain for Reducing Cost of Customized Healthcare System

S. Porkodi** and D. Kesavaraja
Department of Computer Science and Engineering,
Dr. Sivanthi Aditanar College of Engineering,
Tiruchendur, Tamilnadu, India

Abstract

Healthcare is a growing industry in the era of digital technology. Internet of things has been adopted in many big hospitals whereas small customized health care centers don't have much access to technology, thus there is a lack in utilizing the latest innovations. Information retrieval along with data privacy and security is a major concern while developing information retrieval systems, thus blockchain is used. A customized clinical lab information retrieval system is designed by implementing several sensors in the clinic for testing lab results and telemedicine usage. In this chapter, the architecture of an information

* Corresponding Author's E-mail: ishwaryaporkodi6296@gmail.com.

retrieval system for small healthcare centers and clinics is proposed. The system consists of sensors to collect data, an encrypted blockchain cloud gives security and data privacy to create links and transmit data between sensors, and analytical tools are to process, retrieve and evaluate the health condition of the patient. To develop a privacy-preserving e-Health Record with high security, this system deploys a novel blockchain technique with a hybrid algorithm. Business worth is promoted by improving the benefits and minimizing the cost of smart clinical lab information retrieval systems. The goal is to decrease the expenses of the customized healthcare system, retrieve and manage telemedicine data, give high security to patient details and dynamic healthcare data, and improve the efficiency of the outpatient visit.

Keywords: information retrieval system, blockchain, healthcare system, security

INTRODUCTION

Today and Tomorrow

The technological revolution in today's world introduces many new technologies with high potential leading to the development of a better world. Some of the developing technologies include the Internet of Things and Blockchain. In the future, these technologies can be adapted for the development of information retrieval systems, which can also be made to use in clinical laboratories and customized healthcare systems. Thus, the testing process in the lab test and telemedicine are easy and cheaper to perform.

Vision

The major vision is to adapt the Blockchain and Internet of Things technologies to smaller clinical labs and get maximized benefits. The usage of these technologies makes patient data highly secure, manages data, and reduces the expenses of the clinic. Many small clinical centers and small labs can develop their work in these technological areas to sustain longer in the future.

Internet of Things

In the Internet of Things, a thing could be animals with biochip transponders in an animal farm, a human implanted with a heart monitor, a vehicle that is built with a set of sensors to give alert to driver when there is an accident in the same road or a road blockage or even to intimate a tier's low pressure in that vehicle also any man-made or natural objects and devices with a unique IP address are capable of transferring the collected data via the internet. The things can be interconnected to each other, capable of computing on a smaller level and acts as a good communication medium. There are many applications under development based on the Internet of Things because of the ability to adapt to any environment and unique features. IoT devices are becoming more smart and powerful technology (Gillis 2020).

In the developing world, lots of industries increasingly use the Internet of Things to understand the customers better to provide a better service, to improve the operating efficiency, learn and develop the decision-making process also to maximize their business value (Abdulaziz 2019; Dauwed and Ahmed 2019). In this proposed chapter, one such system called clinical lab information system is designed to reduce cost and yield greater benefits by using IoT.

Risks in IoT

The IoT devices are exposed many security issues since they are more physically and virtually vulnerable to attack (Pramanik et al. 2019, 210). The risks in the IoT devices are as shown in Figure 1, attacks at the endpoint (where the IoT devices connect to the internet), unauthorized access, accessing sensitive data, data breaches, and small IoT devices in remote areas are vulnerable to be stolen.

There are other attacks too, such as Denial of Service (DoS) attack, communication channel attack where an attacker could eavesdrop. Network protocol attack such as Sybil attack where device pretending to be authorized device, replay attack, middle man attack, wormhole attack, etc. Software attacks such as back door attacks, viruses, etc. (Porkodi and Kesavaraja 2020a, 79). So, IoT security is much important to protect the system and aspiring businesses. Thus, blockchain with its smart contract and encryption can be used to solve the security issues in IoT devices.

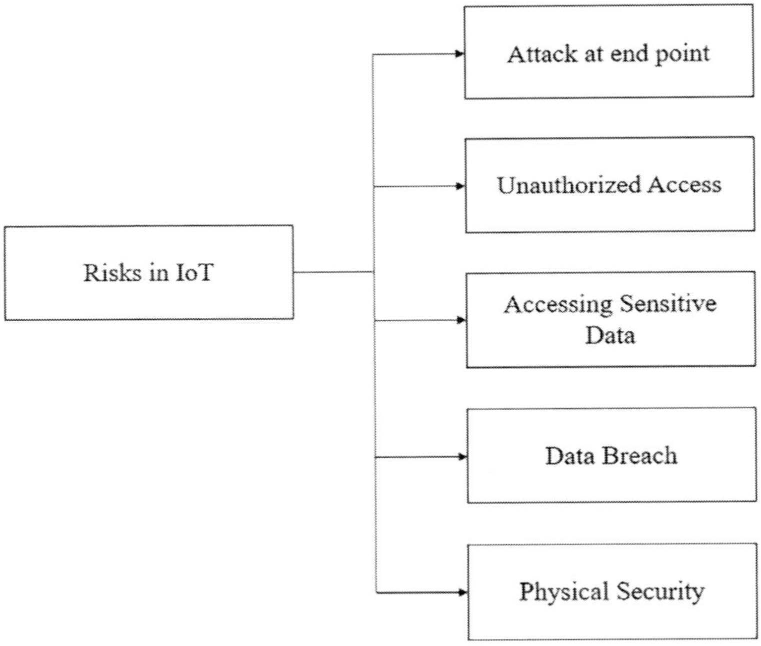

Figure 1. Various risks in the Internet of Things.

Blockchain

The blockchain was initially used for bitcoin transactions by Satoshi Nakamoto in the year 2009 but, it has been evolved. Blockchain is a distributive public digital ledger that would become a new backbone of the internet in near future. It is programmed to record all the transactions with timestamps such as the date and time of transaction along with the transacted amount. The data records within the blockchain known as blocks keep on growing. The digital data blocks are in the public database. The blocks also have the data of the persons who are involved in the transactions, such as sender and receiver details. The blocks are secured with cryptographic encryption (Clauson et al. 2018; Choo et al. 2020). One of the special characteristics of the blockchain is that it has no central authority, which is a decentralized system. To obtain the distributive ledger in blockchain, peer to peer network is used. The major properties of blockchain include anonymity, tamper-resistant, integrity, data security, and privacy (Rosic 2016; Porkodi and Kesavaraja 2020b, 299). The data could be accessed better and faster with low fraud risk (Porkodi and Kesavaraja 2020d, 76).

There are three different types of blockchain that includes public, private, and consortium blockchain. The public blockchain has no central authority, anyone can join the network and the ledger is open to everyone in the network. Whereas the private blockchain is permissioned, has central authority for certain operations in the network, only invited members can join the network and all the ledger content are not open to the nodes of the network. So, the file can be accessed only by authorized members that can be controlled by smart contracts. The consortium blockchain (hybrid blockchain) is also permissioned, has central authority for certain operations in the network, the transparency of the ledger is only given to the selected group of nodes based on the hierarchy of authority over the data. Consortium blockchain could be preferred for the customized healthcare system, since the patients, doctors, physicians can have full access to the patient data. Whereas, the other people in the system could be restricted easily and the researchers can have access only to the medical details and not the patient details. All these different variations could be performed in the hybrid blockchain with the usage of smart contracts and access control policy.

There are lots of applications developed based on Blockchain technology. In this proposed chapter, a clinical lab information system is designed to yield high security, better manageability by using blockchain.

Multi-Sensor System

A single sensor can't be able to reach a comprehensive diagnosis. It is one of the major hindrances to utilize newly developed bio-sensors in the field of medicine. The high rate of the bio-sensor is also a reason, where a single patient can't afford to get a bio-sensor for their treatment. Another problem is that frequent exchange of data during data collection and data analytics process has a huge change to create security failure in handling patient's private information (Biosensors 2021).

These problems can be solved by using secure blockchain technology (Porkodi and Kesavaraja 2020c, 155). The traditional method in the clinic is that a patient has to take a lab test and wait for a few days or weeks for the result. But the usage of a real-time multisensory system replaces the time delay and makes the process much faster. The architecture of the information retrieval system can be seen in Figure 2.

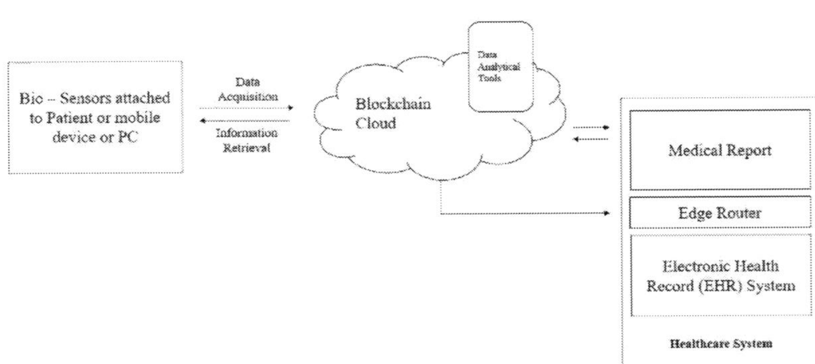

Figure 2. Information Retrieval System Architecture.

In the future, the system can also be extended to create telemedicine applications and even to check the vital signs of patients, which usually needs a long period of monitoring.

SENSORS AND THEIR PARAMETERS

Sensors in healthcare wearable or small devices attached to the patient are used to observe, diagnose, and treat diseases. The medical sensors include a body temperature sensor, glucometer, oximeter, heart rate sensor, Electrocardiogram sensor (ECG), Electroencephalogram sensor, blood pressure sensor, etc.

The traditional laboratory tests have accuracy ranging between 94% and 95.5% (Zweig 1988, 386). The sensors approved by Food and Drug Administration (FDA) are used in the study of this chapter for ensuring accuracy in deduction and analysis of the test results. In the Internet of things laboratory, the accuracy of the sensor ranges from 91% to 99%. The rate of the equipment used in the traditional lab test ranges between ₹75,000 and ₹8, 00,000, which is extremely high. Whereas the rate of the mini biosensors studied in this chapter only cost between ₹5000 and ₹1, 50,000 (Medical 2021).

The results found in the IoT labs are almost equivalent to the results of the traditional lab. But the cost of the biosensors is found much cheaper than the traditional equipment used for the lab tests in the clinic. So the cost can be highly decreased by using biosensors in clinical laboratories.

ARCHITECTURE OF THE INFORMATION RETRIEVAL SYSTEM

The backbone of the Internet of things sensor labs will be the system with blockchain-based architecture. This system mainly enables communication among sensors and also keeps the data secure during the process of data retrieval and the data transfer process. It also maintains the privacy of the sensitive and personal data of the users (Subramanian 2021). There are two types of data they are, data in motion and data in rest. Data in motion or data in flight are the data moving between different locations across the internet and the private network. Data in rest are the data which is been stored in a single device or any network.

Both types of data are secured by robust encryption mechanisms in the traditional method of data security. The encryption mechanism includes verification between actions. The usage of blockchain technology removes the necessity of the trusted middleman third party and the organization's auditing capability is enhanced for the identification of the threats in the system. The biggest and costliest threat to the information systems at the hospital or clinic is the intrusion or someone gaining access to the systems and causing problems, lack or deleting security to cause harm. The Digital Ledger Technology (DLT) of the blockchain is termed as auditing logs, which addresses the weakness in modifying the blocks or records by using the system agreement. In addition to this, the record management systemically enhances the analysis, threat, or intrusion deduction tools like anomalies detection. To make the system much more consistent, norms are established in the behavior of the system (Mafli 2017), and finding deviations becomes much easier.

Data Transmission and Information Retrieval in E-Health Record

In the Internet of Things sensor lab, there already exists E-Health Record (EHR) system which is intergraded with a private blockchain cloud. Many EHR systems are offered as Software as a service (SaaS) model along with capabilities of IoT, which later can easily be implemented in small health care centers and small clinics.

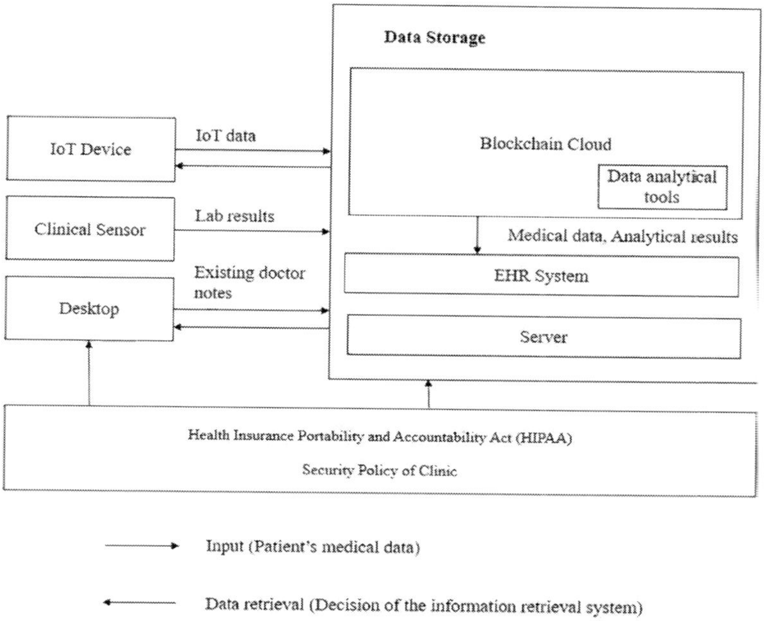

Figure 3. Data Transmission and Information Retrieval in E-Health Record System.

The advantages of the blockchain in the EHR systems are secured accounts integrity, maintenance of data and files security, efficient monitoring, and management of all the health care data accurately. The medical records need extra storage since they can't be placed on the blockchain cloud as they can be globally visible. But blockchain cloud can be used to save the temporary sensor data, which is waiting to be transferred. The primary purpose of the blockchain is to connect all the IoT devices and then transfers the data to the EHR system. The data flow process to the E-Health Record system can be seen in Figure 3.

A protocol called Enigma Protocol, which uses the open blockchain to do auditing, identity management, and access control process. This protocol mainly describes privacy for programmable substrate, which is used to share secrets and provide security to multiparty computation to achieve complete Turing computation of the private data. The usual check-in process of the clinic or private key is used to perform identity management.

To integrate sensors within the Cloud and to the EHR system, Smart Contracts are used in Ethereum (Solidity 2021). The existing medical data and records are stored in a location from which the cryptographic instructions perform read and write operations on the data only in the existing system. To integrate sensor lab into the existing system, few contracts are necessary, they are listed below.

Types of Contracts

- Registrar Contract: It gives unique identification IDs to the EHR address of the patient.
- Patient – Admin Contract: In the system patient–admin contract is between the patient, who provides details for the system, and the admin, who stores the provided information and manages it for identifying the records whenever necessary. In addition, the contract explains various data pointers and its access rights permission that is used to identify records that are stored with the admin database. Every pointer has a query string attached to a hash. The hash returns the patient's data subset during the time of execution in the database of admin. Each separate sensor will have its separate own pointer. This process gives assurance that the details of the patients are not modified in the database without the approval of the patient.
- Summary Contract: It is a trial to locate the sensor data of the patients and to give summary analytics. This contract provides patient–admin contract reference list along with user notification (Yuan, Wendy and Colin 2016).

Cloud and Security

The data of the sensor can be hashed using cryptography, this process can prevent data tampering since permission is necessary to view the data. Data shared among admins are authorized and permitted by the patients. This cryptographic hashing assures the integrity of the data and security of the system by proof of work during the communication between sensor and EHR system. It provides a trustless distributed consensus within the nodes of the systems (Bulkin 2016). Strong cryptographic techniques like Ciphertext Policy Using Blowfish Hybridized Weighted Attribute-Based Encryption (Porkodi and Kesavaraja 2021a, 108; Porkodi and Kesavaraja 2021b, 204; Wang and Juntao 2018) can be used in the blockchain chain where the nodes in the network are assigned with weights to their attributes and are used during encryption along with the access rights policy.

Patient data is not stored in any private cloud, but it serves as a medium in between the EHR system and the Internet of Things sensor lab. Not only the sensor data communication happens over the cloud but also does the data analytics and gives the analyzed data to the summary contract where it produces summary analytics of patients directly. The live data from the sensors are only stored temporarily and analytical summaries or results are stored permanently for a long time in the existing patient's record. A patient can verify identity themselves in the cloud by using public key encryption while entering the sensor lab this is used to enable the verified patient's session and later terminated automatically when the patient exits the sensor lab.

User Interface of Patients for Information Retrieval

All the biosensors which are based on PC are connected to a single PC. The majority of the biosensors which are very small in size are mostly cell phone-based so they can be mounted onto the smartphone. The data that is collected from every sensor in the IoT sensor lab is then directed to the EHR system. In the EHR system, the data are analyzed based on the patient's existing data. Analytical methodologies that are based on machine learning transfer the important health information to the blockchain cloud, in which the patient can access the statistics of the summary by using their own cell phones.

Analytics of Data

When the combination of the sensors is optimal for all the patients, it will lead to different datasets. There are various sources in which data is generated, each data source has some principal conditions. Even if a single parameter went out of the range, it can be found easily in the result. The reason for this is mostly a benign condition or the sensor has to be budged. If there arises any dangerous set of situation, it will be notified to the physician, this action may add additional value to some random data. Then the analytics is been carried out for specific disease levels and also diseases that are correlated.

Patients with more than three chronic conditions utilize this system highly. It is found to be 96% whereas 20% of the adults are from the U.S. are found to have more than two chronic conditions. The patient's chronic conditions can be identified by the EHR system and classify the risk of the patients based on the different chronic conditions. The EHR system consists of admin data, ICD – 10 code for diagnosis, medications, charts, and clinical notes. To perform analytics, only a limited number of dataset items are used excluding the personal contents of the patients which are to be protected such as their name, address (except district, state, and pin code), fax number, cell phone number, Social Security Number (SSN) or Aadhar Number or any personal user identification numbers, Email ID, medical record management number, payment account details, health beneficiary plans number, vehicle or license details, certificates details, Internet protocol (IP) and Universal resource locator (URL) address, Biometric details (such as voice, fingerprints and face recognition) and any other comparable pictures.

To stream the acquired data a platform is needed, which can absorb the collected data with the bandwidth that can handle many different waveforms in many different fidelities. Analytics of data is to enrich the data to necessary information it makes the system much more robust, to do prediction analysis and balance sensitivity of data.

To perform analytics on telemetry continuous waveform, the Apache Spark is been integrated into the Hadoop stack. Because this integration can absorb the collected data and do computation on the data with the help of graphing tools and machine learning. Coding is required for both online analysis and batch mode analyzing which, requires large RAM to process. MongoDB is a document-oriented cross-platform open-source database independent of the table-based traditional database (Medical 2021).

Consensus-based or fault-tolerant strategies are implemented mainly to handle data crowdsourcing which is when a huge set of patients submit data through the internet. All the irrelevant data are cleaned, repairs data or can combine any operators for data integration by using outlier detection. Several models of the sensor can be used to carry out unsupervised phenotyping (Richesson 2016, 60). There are some disadvantages in the unsupervised techniques are,

- The phenotypes sometimes overlap with one another.
- The existing knowledge of the doctor should still be integrated manually.
- The phenotypes are much large-sized and with large dimensions and so high scalability is required (Wang et al. 2015, 1272).

Combine the dynamic data with the static data of the EHR system is a big challenge but it provides contextual and situational insights. Since the symptoms of the patient evolve in time, thus the semantics and dimension of data overlap. This approach turns like a crowdsourcing entry in that many parts of patient data have to give a contribution to the conditions of certain diseases which is monitored frequently after diagnosing. The records are arranged based on the priority of metrics and then they are added into the priority queue. When the queue is called iteratively based on the disease the entity resolution solutions are given based on the clustering algorithm (Gruenheid 2016).

When a machine is once trained based on the machine learning algorithm then to diagnose and predict conclusions from it. Further, the doctor or physician can deliver the prescription to the patients easily. It can also explain the parameters meaning for primary health care which is need for certain specialties (such as more accurate reference and diagnosis is a need in specialty areas like brain wave, EKG, EMG, etc. to understand the results of analytics better) (Szlosek and Jonathan 2016).

Clinical Lab Information System as Business Model

General Partnership

The streaming of data in real-time may appear to be simple but the sensor company's cooperation may get complex since in the future there may be a requirement to see the past recorded history of the patients. In case of that, a general partnership has to be signed to send the patient's sensor data from the cloud to a private data storage area. Insured of a joint venture, a general partnership is preferred as it needs no utilization of personal income tax, to allow shares in the business profit and there are many more feasible also valuable advantages. But in the EHR system integration, there are some limits in commercialization such as the usage of the dataset is limited for the use of public health, research purpose, and health care system operations.

Field Hospitals vs Critical Access Hospitals

The Internet of Things sensor system labs could be used in hospitals or health care with insufficient equipment. Critical access hospitals are hospitals with only fewer labs and equipment. There are more critical access hospitals even in 2016. The Internet of Things sensor lab also can be used in field hospitals, military medical camps, and health care near combats in a foreign country. A minimum deployment of IoT sensor lab can be done in case of medical emergencies of civilians.

Practices in Value-Based Primary Care

The majority of lab tests are purchased mainly by primary health care providers. In the total, 800 million lab visits nearly half of the visits to physicians in the office are due to primary health care practices, including family and general visits (25%), pediatrics visits (13%), and internal medicine (15%) (Richesson et al. 2016, 60; Bernstein 2004). The benefits of the clinics with a value-based care system are they improve inaccurate diagnostics with fast and wide-ranging data collected from the sensor, even data analytics cover some of the specialty areas. The sensor lab can be used without the marginal cost incurred. Thus in the payment based on value modifier, the factor of saving cost can be seen. The payment based on value modifier on health care is imposed to a group of more than ten physicians around 2016, after 2016 it was reduced to a group of more than two physicians. A pay of +4% incentive or -4% penalty is given to a group of more than ten physicians and −2% incentive or -2% penalty is given to a group of more than two physicians. The health care benefits and physician's visit to the office counts around half of the total clinic visits. The traditional testing existing equipment in the clinic like Glucometer, INR test machine, EKG, urinalysis, rapid strep test machine are replaced in sensor lab. The clinic with traditional equipment expenses a total cost is much huge than the clinics with sensors.

This can be applied to more than 30, 000 primary health care clinics in 2013 and also more than 9,000 urgent health care centers with sensor labs which are located in the United States (Census 2021; Lozier 2021). Conventional complex methods for checking bacterial or yeast infection can be found only under the microscope in the traditional clinic, which is replaced by sensors that operate in few seconds. Delay in digenesis may lead to maximize the medical cost losing several thousand for a single patient, it also leads to chances of malpractice (Suszek 2015). If a patient has taken insurance then an incentive is paid in such situations as medical costs.

Conclusion

The Internet of Things clinical multi-sensor lab information system is capable of providing a more comprehensive, efficient, and potential diagnosis. The IoT clinical lab information system monitors the real-time health of the patient's condition with the help of sensors and data analytics devices. Every patient has a customized set of biosensors based on the health condition of the patient. To interpret all the parameters, analytics based on machine learning is used. Using IoT sensor labs can completely minimize the waiting time of patients and sensor lab can give much faster results than the traditional labs which takes much time to produce results. The personal information of patients is secretly sent via blockchain cloud, which is then saved in the EHR system of the client, this process requires three contracts to be signed. The patients can verify their identity themselves in the cloud through public-key encryption.

Internet of Things multisensory clinical lab information system is implemented to provide value-based care by primary health care clinics so they can get little incentives for their care. As the traditional equipment is been replaced by sensors in the IoT sensor lab, the cost of getting and maintaining the technology is highly reduced also the delay in diagnoses and malpractices are completely reduced. The public health planners or authorities can also get better details about general public health. The IoT sensor's data flow is analyzed to get health surveillance.

References

Abdulaziz Albesher. (2019). "IoT in Health-care: Recent Advances in the Development of Smart Cyber-Physical Ubiquitous Environment." *IJCSNS International Journal of Computer Science and Network Security*, *19*(2), 181-186.

Bernstein, Amy. (2004). *Health Care in America; Trends in Utilization*. Accessed May 18, 2021. https://stacks.cdc.gov/ view/cdc/11299.

Biosensors. (2021). *Overview.* Accessed May 18. https://www.biosensors.com/intl/clinical-program.

Bulkin, Aleksandr. (2016). *Explaining Blockchain — How Proof of Work Enables Trustless Consensus.* Last modified May 3. https://keepingstock.net/explaining-blockchain-how-proof-of-work-enables-trustless-consensus-2abed27f0845.

Census. (2021). *Ambulatory Health Care Services Receipts and Employment on the Upswing, According to Census Bureau's Economic Census.* Accessed May 19. https://www.census.gov/newsroom/press-releases/2014/cb14-216.html.

Choo, Kim-Kwang Raymond, Ali Dehghantanha. & Reza M. Parizi. eds. (2020). *Blockchain Cybersecurity, Trust and Privacy.* 1st ed. Cham, Switzerland: Springer Nature.

Clauson, Kevin A., Elizabeth A. Breeden, Cameron Davidson. & Timothy K. Mackey. (2018). "Leveraging Blockchain Technology to Enhance Supply Chain Management in Healthcare: An Exploration of Challenges and Opportunities in the Health Supply Chain." *Blockchain in Healthcare Today.* doi:10.30953/bhty.v1.20.

Dauwed, Mohammed. & Ahmed Meri. (2019). "IOT Service Utilisation in Healthcare." In *IoT and Smart Home Automation [Working Title]*, edited by Yasser Ismail. London, England: IntechOpen. Accessed May 19.

Gillis, Alexander S. (2020). *What Is IoT (Internet of Things) and How Does It Work?* Accessed February 11, 2021. https://internetofthingsagenda.techtarget.com/definition/Internet-of-Things-IoT.

Gruenheid, Anja. (2016). "Data Integration with Dynamic Data Sources." *ETH Zurich.*

Lozier institute. (2021) *Maps: Health Clinics Nationwide Compared to Planned Parenthood Centers.* Accessed May 19. https://lozierinstitute.org/health-clinics-nationwide-compared-to-planned-parenthood-centers/.

Mafli, Ken. (2017). *Mega Data Breaches Could Drive the Blockchain Revolution.* Last modified May 1. https:// www.infosecurity-magazine.com/opinions/data-breaches-Blockchain-revolution/.

Medical Price Online. (2021). *Clinical Lab*. Accessed May 18. https://www.medicalpriceonline.com/medical-equipment/clinical-lab/.

Porkodi, S. & Kesavaraja, D. (2020a). "Integration of Blockchain and Internet of Things." In *Handbook of Research on Blockchain Technology*, edited by Saravanan Krishnan, Valentina E. Balas, E. Golden Julie, Y. Harold Robinson, S. Balaji, and Raghvendra Kumar, 61–94. San Diego, CA: Elsevier.

Porkodi, S. & Kesavaraja, D. (2020b). "A Trust-based Recommender System Built on IoT Blockchain Network with Cognitive Framework." *Recommender System with Machine Learning and Artificial Intelligence: Practical Tools and Applications in Medical, Agricultural and Other Industries*., 291-311. John Wiley & Sons, Inc. doi:10.1002/9781119711582.ch15.

Porkodi, S. & Kesavaraja, D. (2020c). "8. Smart Health Care Service Evolution with Internet of Things." In *Predictive Intelligence in Biomedical and Health Informatics*, vol. *2*, 145–64. De Gruyter.

Porkodi, S. & Kesavaraja, D. (2020d). "Blockchain in Healthcare Sector." In *Bitcoin and Blockchain*, 163–82. Boca Raton, FL: CRC Press.

Porkodi, S. & Kesavaraja, D. (2021a). "Secure Ciphertext Policy Using Blowfish Hybridized Weighted Attribute-Based Encryption." In *Advances in Smart System Technologies*, 103–17. Singapore: Springer Singapore.

Porkodi, S. & Kesavaraja, D. (2021b). "Safe & Secure Ciphertext Policy Attribute Based Encryption to Avoid Suicidal Games Nn Entering Whatsapp or Mobile like Bluewhale Game or Momo Challenge." *International Journal of Research in Advent Technology (IJRAT)*., 201-206. Accessed May 19.

Pramanik, Pijush Kanti Dutta, Gaurav Pareek. & Anand Nayyar. (2019). "Security and Privacy in Remote Healthcare." In *Telemedicine Technologies*, edited by Hemanth D. Jude and Valentina Emilia Balas, 201–25. San Diego, CA: Elsevier.

Richesson, Rachel L., Jimeng Sun, Jyotishman Pathak, Abel N. Kho. & Joshua C. Denny. (2016). "Clinical Phenotyping in Selected National Networks: Demonstrating the Need for High-Throughput, Portable, and Computational Methods." *Artificial Intelligence in Medicine*, *71*, 57–61.

Rosic, Ameer. (2016). *What Is Blockchain Technology? A Step-by-Step Guide for Beginners.* Accessed February 11, 2021. https://blockgeeks.com/guides/what-is-blockchain-technology/.

Solidity. (2021). *Introduction to Smart Contracts — Solidity 0.8.5 Documentation.* Accessed May 18. https://solidity.readthedocs.io/en/develop/introduction-to-smart-contracts.html.

Subramanian Iyer. (2021). *The Benefits of Blockchain across Industries.* Accessed May 18 https://blogs.oracle.com/profit/the-benefits-of-blockchain-across-industries.

Suszek, Andrew. (2015). *Medical Malpractice: Misdiagnosis and Failure to Diagnose.* Last modified March 10. https:// www.alllaw.com/articles/nolo/medical-malpractice/delayed-diagnosis.html.

Szlosek, Donald A. & Jonathan Ferrett. (2016). "Using Machine Learning and Natural Language Processing Algorithms to Automate the Evaluation of Clinical Decision Support in Electronic Medical Record Systems." *EGEMS* (Washington, DC), *4* (3), 1222.

Wang, Yichen, Robert Chen, Joydeep Ghosh, Joshua C. Denny, Abel Kho, You Chen, Bradley A. Malin. & Jimeng Sun. (2015). "Rubik: Knowledge Guided Tensor Factorization and Completion for Health Data Analytics." *International Conference on Knowledge Discovery & Data Mining. International Conference on Knowledge Discovery & Data Mining*, 1265–74. doi:10.1145/ 2783258.2783395.

Wang, Yuxiao. & Juntao Gao. (2018). "A Regulation Scheme Based on the Ciphertext-Policy Hierarchical Attribute-Based Encryption in Bitcoin System." *IEEE Access: Practical Innovations, Open Solutions*, *6*, 16267–78.

Yuan, Ben, Wendy Lin. & Colin McDonnell. (2016). *Blockchains and electronic health records*. Mcdonnell. mit. Edu.

Zweig, M. H. (1988). "Evaluation of the Clinical Accuracy of Laboratory Tests." *Archives of Pathology & Laboratory Medicine*, *112* (4), 383–86. Accessed February 11, 2021.

About the Authors

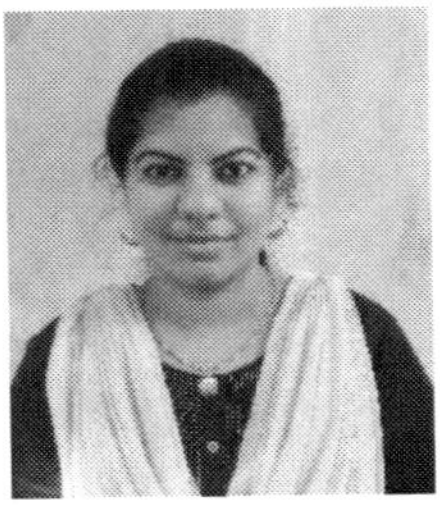

S. Porkodi was born in 1996, she has completed her Master Degree in department of Computer Science and Engineering in Dr. Sivanthi Aditanar College of Engineering, Tiruchendur in May 2019. She has Received a fund of Rs.4000 Grand cash for her PG project titled "Safe and secure ciphertext policy attribute based encryption to avoid suicidal games on entering whatsapp or mobile like bluewhale game or momo challenge" from Tamilnadu State Council for Science and Technology (TNSCST) under student project scheme 2018-2019. She has Won Best Paper Work Award for "Secure Cipher Text Blowfish Hybridized Weighted Attribute Based Encryption" in fourth National Conference on innovative Computing Techniques and Applications (NCICTA'19) held at VV College of Engineering, Tisayanvillai. She has published two International Journal, three International and six National conference works. Her research interests are Network Security, Cryptography, Blockchain and Internet of Things.

E-mail: Ishwaryaporkodi6296@gmail.com

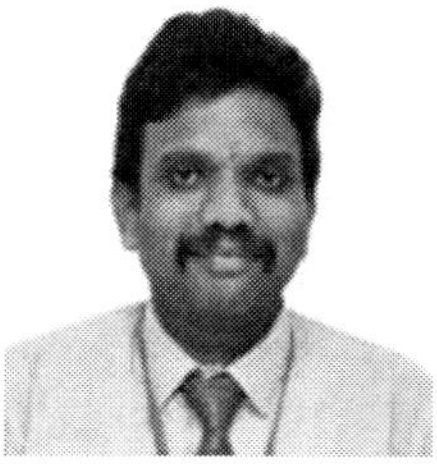

D. Kesavaraja is working as an Associate Professor, Department of CSE, Dr. Sivanthi Aditanar College of Engineering, Tiruchendur. He has 14 years and 11 months of Teaching Experience. He has completed his B.E (CSE) from Jayaraj Annapackiam CSI College of Engineering, Nazareth under Anna University Chennai in 2005, M.E (CSE) from Manonmaniam Sundaranar University, Tirunelveli in 2010 and Ph.D (Cloud Computing) from Anna University, Chennai in April 2019. He is a co-author of a book titled "Fundamentals of Computing and Programming" and "Fundamentals of LaTeX Programming" and published 3 Book Chapters (Elsevier & IGI Global). He received SAP Award of Excellence from IIT Bombay and Outstanding Reviewer Award from Elsevier Computers & Electrical Engineering Journal. He has published many National and International Journal and conference papers. He is a recognized PhD supervisor for Anna University, Chennai. He has served as a reviewer for scientific journals such as Springer, Elsevier, IET, T&F and Technical Programme Committee Member for International Conferences. He has guided 2 student R&D Projects Sponsored by IE (I), Kolkatta and TNSCST. He presented 145 seminars and workshops. He has presented Two International webinars (MAHSA University, Malaysia & DMI – ST.JOHN THE BAPTIST UNIVERSITY, Malawi). His research interests include Cloud Computing, Internet of Things, Machine Learning and Blockchain Technology. More information at http://www.k7cloud.in

E-mail: dkeasavaraja@gmail.com

In: Intelligent Information Retrieval … ISBN: 978-1-68507-301-5
Editors: Parma Nand et al. © 2021 Nova Science Publishers, Inc.

Chapter 2

ONTOLOGICAL MULTI-AGENT SYSTEM FOR PANDEMIC ZONE CLASSIFICATION AND AUTOMATED POLICY FORMULATION

Gaurav Kant Shankhdhar[1,*], Himanshu Pandey[2,†], M. Darbari[3,‡], Anurag Tiwari[4,§] and Bhaskar Karn[5]

[1]Department of Mathematics and Computer Science, Babu Banarasi Das University, Lucknow, India

[2]Faculty of Engineering and Technology, University of Lucknow, Lucknow, Uttar Pradesh, India

[3]Department of IT, Babu Banarasi Das National Institute of Technology and Management, Lucknow, India, Sr.Member, IEEE

[4]Department of IT, Babu Banarasi Das National Institute of Technology and Management, Lucknow, India

[5]Department of Computer Science and Engineering, Birla Institute of Technology, Mesra, Ranchi

[*] Corresponding Author's E-mail: g.kant.82@gmail.com.

[†] Corresponding Author's E-mail: hpandey010@gmail.com.

[‡] Corresponding Author's E-mail: manuj_darbari@acm.org.

[§] Corresponding Author's E-mail: anuragrktiwari@gmail.com.

ABSTRACT

This chapter deals with in depth analysis and design of a multi-agent system supported by a thorough knowledge base, Covid19_ONT, developed and enriched in Protégé 5.2.0. NLP is used to extract the information regarding COVID-19 from valuable sources like mygov.in, who.int, nhs.uk and others. India introduced the concept of zones according to the degree and magnitude of the disease. The red, orange and green zones were demarcated through the districts at the lowest level. A district at any time can be in one of the zones and it is also possible that the district might wave between the zones according to the number of active cases. Each of the zones has its own rules to be imposed, called policies. This chapter allows for systematic allotment of zones to the districts and automated policy formulation for the districts by using ontological inference done through the Drool's reasoner.

INTRODUCTION

The corona virus COVID-19 [1, 2] pandemic is the most calamitous and debilitating global health, social, economical and political crisis and the greatest challenge we have faced since World War Two. The pandemic is confronting like a wave that is crashing on the whole human race irrespective of the national boundaries pulling even the most powerful on to his knees. This ruthless phenomenon moves from nation to nation recurring in its proceedings. The only possibility to deal with such a crisis is to take lessons from the countries in which it has occurred and devise measures that can, if any, prove to be fruitful.

Natural Language Processing (NLP) research incorporated Semantic web resources as domain knowledge, and incrementally graph-based methods are entering the realm of semantic tools [3, 4]. Contemporarily, more tools are emerging that involve a deeper KE, typically by hybridizing statistical and rule-based methods, and leveraging existing knowledge from Linked Open Data as well as of smart heuristics that become incrementally available on the Web [5]. One of the extensively used tools is Protégé and its OntoGraph. Protégé comes in varied versions [6, 7]. The authors have used Protégé 5.2.0 as it clubs together tremendously useful tools like

GraphViz, Drools reasoner, OntoGraph and an excellent IDE for ontology creation, enrichment, ontology merging, visualization and inferencing [9, 10].

Traditionally, NLP tasks are distinguished into basic (e.g., named entity recognition), and applied (e.g., question answering). When we try to reuse NLP algorithms for the Semantic Web, we can also distinguish between basic (e.g., class induction) and application tasks (NL querying of linked data) [11, 12].

Software agents are intelligent, autonomous, situated and proactive software entities along with other notable features that can collaborate with other agents in order to perform a job in dynamic environment. They follow the principles of reinforcement learning. They continuously update their beliefs through percepts received by their environment [13, 14].

In order for the MAS to function appropriately they must share a common knowledge base, formally called an ontology [15]. All the agents adhere to the domain concepts held by the ontology.

There are a number of Agent Oriented Software Engineering methodologies available for developing a MAS. These include TROPOS, GORMAS, ROMAS, GAIA, MaSE, O-MaSE and many others. The authors have followed O-MaSE methodologies in order to develop the MAS for pandemic zone classification and policy formulation for COVID-19 [16, 17].

Analysis and Design of Ontological MAS for COVID-19

For the purpose of designing an autonomous system for zone classification and policy formulation the authors first identified the factors that are related to the pandemic [18]. These factors are diagrammatically shown in Figure 1.

All the identified factors may be affected by the COVID-19 fight by India, or these factors will affect the COVID-19 fight [19, 20]. In many cases this effect will be bidirectional.

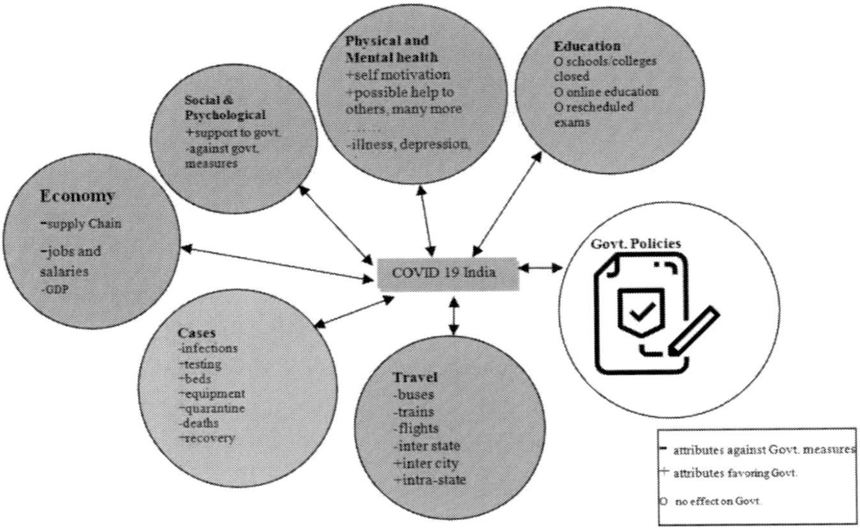

Figure 1. Factors related to COVID-19.

This effect is caused by the attributes of the identified factors. As an instance, case is a factor and no. of infections, tests, beds, deaths, etc. are attributes shown by either +, - or O.

- The change in the values of the attributes of those factors will decide the traversal of the corona spread and its zones.
- These values of the attributes of factors are a result through the government policies and the level of obeying and adherence to these policies by the public.
- It is through this dynamism that a town or a city falls in Red, Orange and Green zone.
- Taking Uttarakhand as an example, first the cases grew to reach the red zone then due the enactment of Govt. measures and various factors contributing in favor of the fight against corona, fewer cases emerged and till now many spots got in the green zone [21].
- Stating in the terms of the ecosystem, the change in the values of the attributes collectively triggered the change in zones.

- The whole COVID-19 is an incredibly dynamic process and extremely strict adherence to the government policies along with tremendous support from public in many ways is needed as experienced from the states that have fought successfully against Corona at least till now.

The Figure 2 below shows the mind map of the whole COVID-19 process faced by India and its containment process involving the three zones.

SOFTWARE AGENTS DEVELOPMENT

The Knowledge Extractor Agent enables to extract information related to COVID-19 from varied sources having the corpus involving the pandemic. Information such as frequency of infected people, active cases, mortality and recovery rate was easily accessible through the data imported from mygov.in, who.int and other sites. But, the data concerning the policies that were enacted to fight against the virus in countries all over the world could only be drawn out through some knowledge extraction mechanism. This is done by using the NLP to identify the named entities and appropriate knowledge elements as shown in Figure 3, KEAgent is built for this purpose.

The overall process of zone classification and policy formulation can be described as Natural language Processing, Knowledge Extraction in the form of annotations, ontology population, enrichment of ontology COVID19_ONT and reasoning. The whole process is shown in Figure 3. In the MAS, the first task, i.e., knowledge extraction is done by the KEAgent by dividing the corpus text into sentences and words. This task was accomplished using GATE (General Architecture for Text Engineering), a framework for NLP [22]. The knowledge extraction for identifying annotations, two of the GATE components JAPE (Java Annotation Patterns Engine) and Gazetteer were used [23].

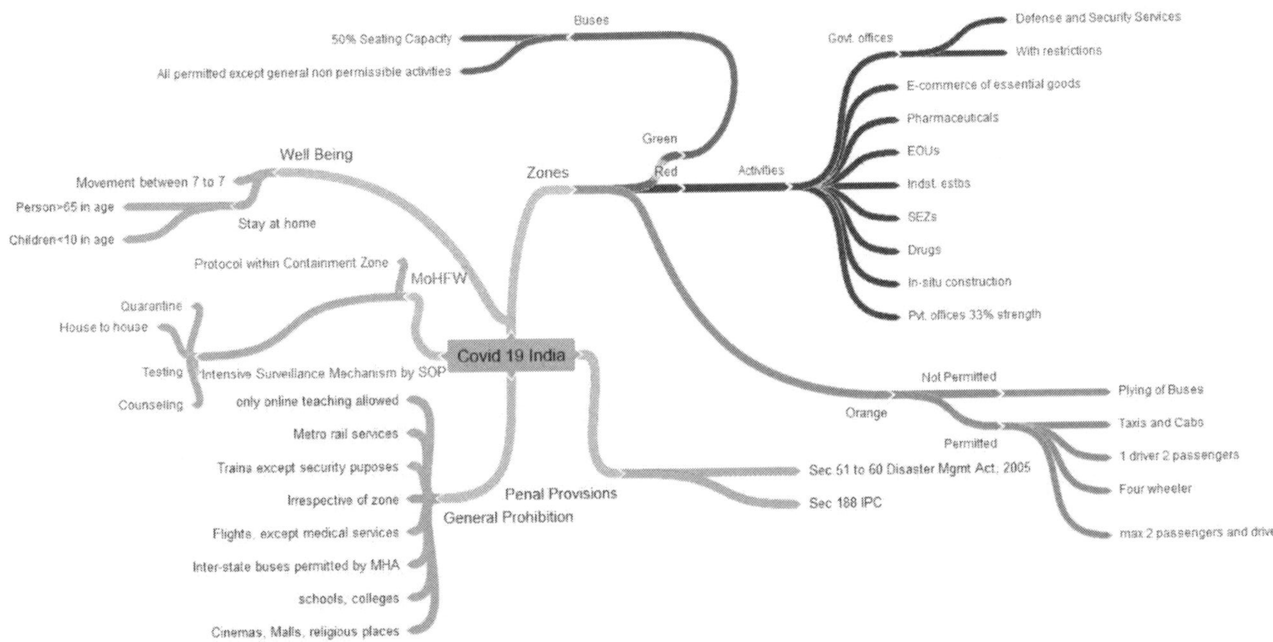

Figure 2. COVID-19 Mindmap.

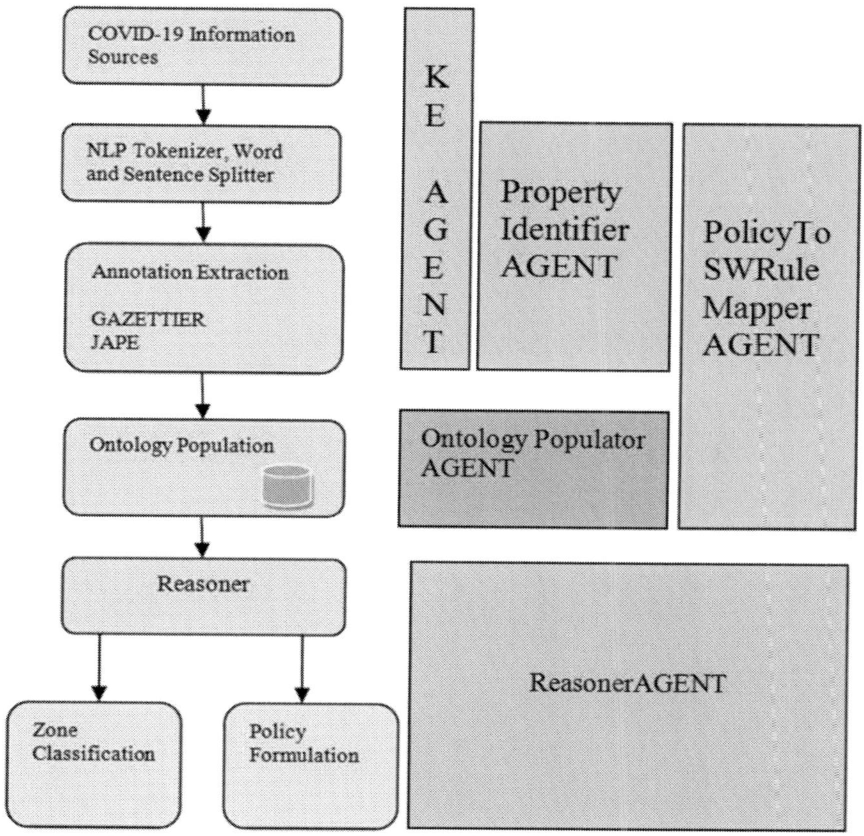

Figure 3. MAS for Zone Classification and Policy Formulation.

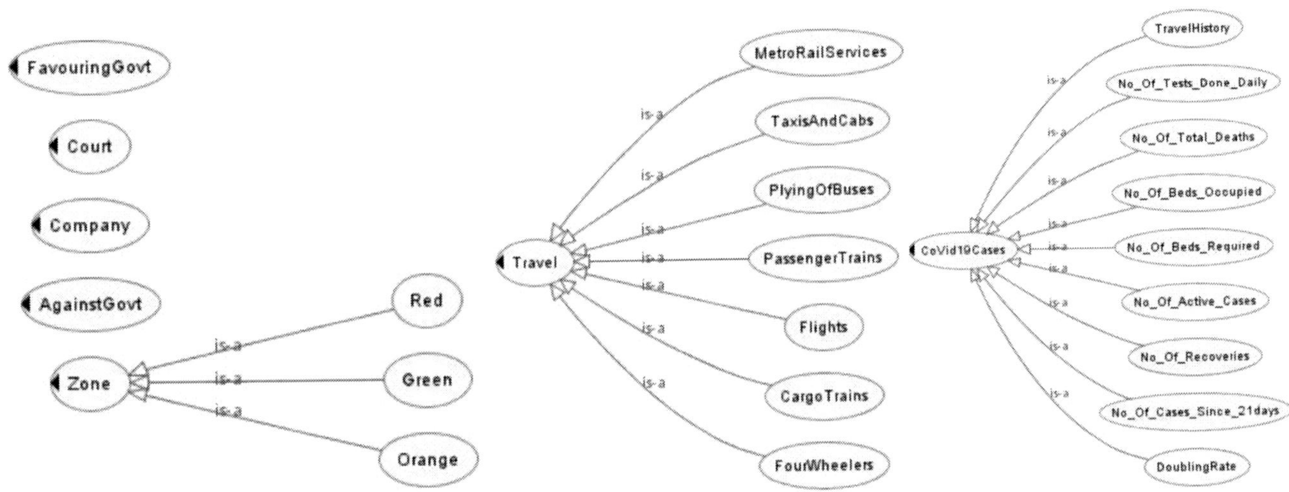

Figure 4a. (Continued)

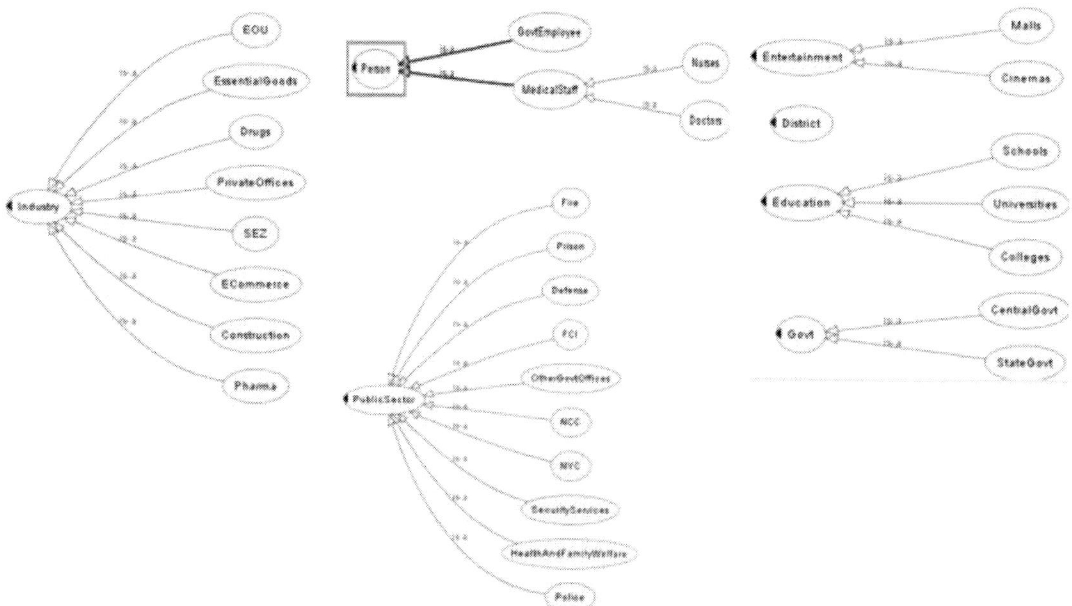

Figure 4a. OwlViz class diagram showing classes extracted by the KEAgent and populated in the COVID19_ONT by the OntologyPopulatorAgent.

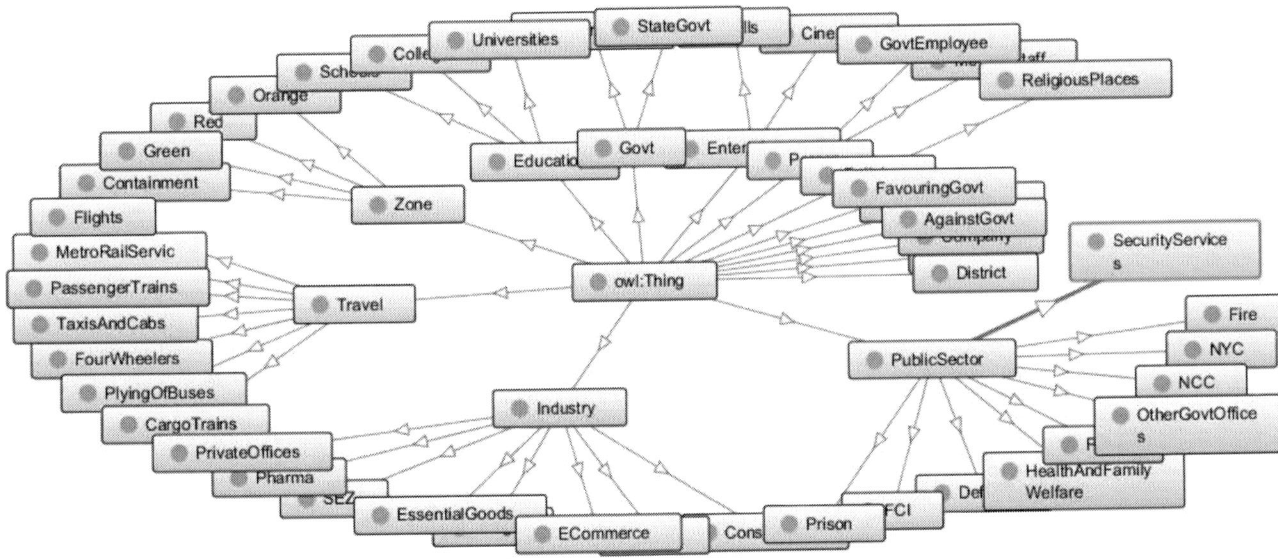

Figure 4b. Protégé OntoGraph class diagram showing classes extracted by the KEAgent and populated in the COVID19_ONT by the OntologyPopulatorAgent.

IMPLEMENTATION OF THE MODEL USING ONTOLOGYPOPULATORAGENT

This phase the objects or individuals as they are called in Protégé are inserted and once the basic structure of the ontology is designed, the annotations extracted by the KEAgent are used to instantiate and enrich the ontology. Figure 4a and 4b shows the class hierarchy of the created COVID19_ONT domain ontology [24].

In order to identify properties the PropertyIdentifierAgent has to search through the policies framed in fight against COVID-19 by Indian Government. The policies are of the following primary types:

Social Policies

Social policies are the policies that have to be followed by the people as a whole. A person who follows the social policies favors and assists government in the fight against COVID-19. People who do not abide to these policies always remain a loophole for Corona fight and can give birth to turmoil and stigma and are categorized as violators.

The social and psychological policies can be diagrammatically represented before putting into some formal language, like SWRL as given below. The identified properties like has Sound Mental Health and is Self Motivated can either be in favor or against as a COVID-19 related factor as shown in Figure 5 in the form of Interaction Protocol Diagram. The process of property assignment can be assisted by the user [25, 26].

Zone Selection Policies

The Indian Government divided the districts amongst red, orange and green zones on the basis of the conditions as given by the figure below.

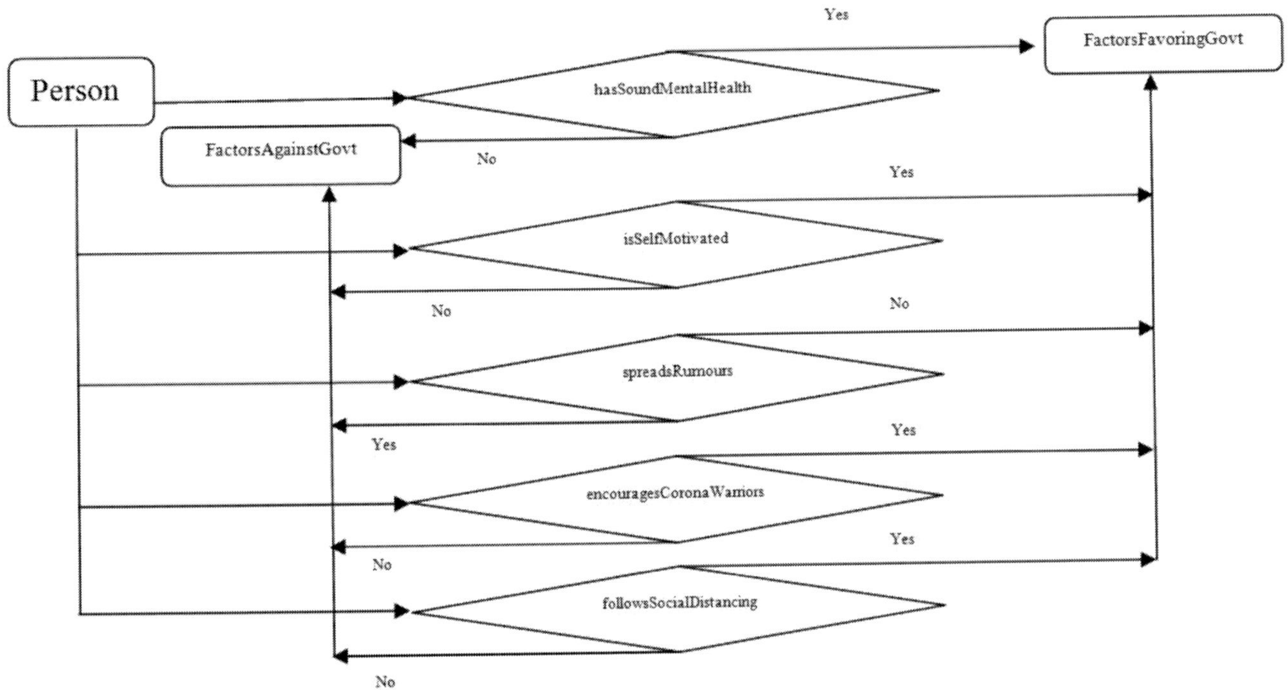

Figure 5. Social and Psychological Properties.

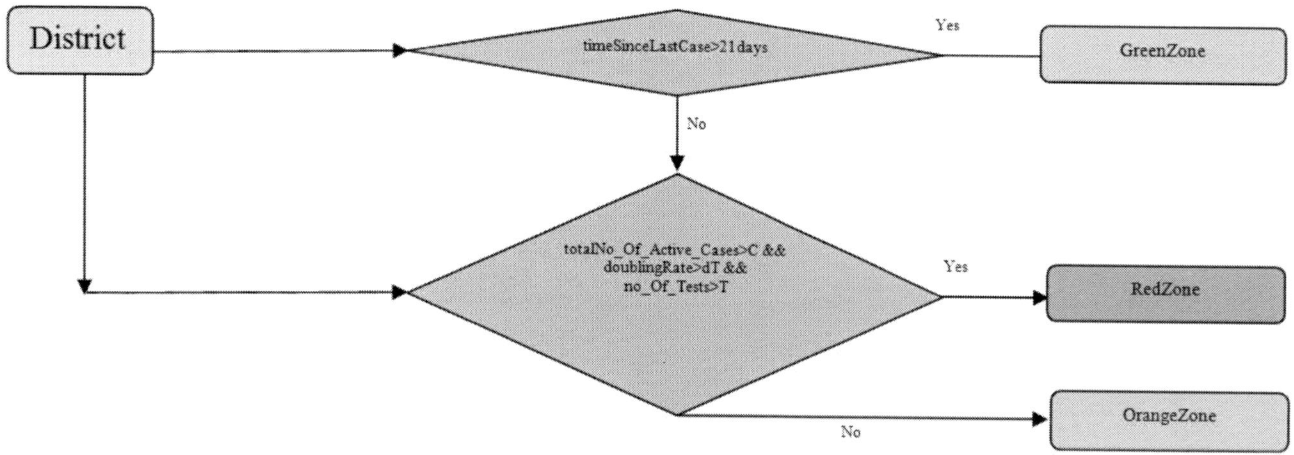

Figure 6. Properties related to Zone selection.

The above figure shows dynamic transformation and selection of zones in districts is difficult to manage by human efforts. The government lays down the conditions for a district to be in any zone which is applied to all the towns and districts in a nation. Once, the conditions are specified for zone allotment then what is needed is a system that is intelligent enough to be able to know and judge all the districts and towns in terms of their zone allotment, social and psychological and legal polices [27], severity level and magnitude of the pandemic at any time.

Containment Policies

The properties identified during containment are centered on contact tracing, quarantining, testing, complete lockdown and proper counseling shown in Figure 7a.

It represents various industries and sectors that would be directly or indirectly affected by the Corona pandemic are identified by KEAgent and then the PropertyIdentifierAgent assigns the has Precaution And Prohibition and level Of Permission properties to the Travel, Education, Industry, Entertainment and other classes.

As can be shown in Figure 7b, the precaution and prohibition is maximum in red zone, medium in orange zone and general in green zone. Similarly, level Of Permission is 'restricted' in red zone [28].

Penal Provisions and Legal Policies [29, 30]

Any person violating the lockdown measures and the National Directives for COVID-19 Management will be liable to be proceeded against as per the provisions of Section 51 to 60 of the Disaster Management Act, 2005, besides legal action under Sec. 188 of the IPC, and other legal provisions as applicable. Through the legal corpus, the Property Identifier Agent is able to identify properties like obstructs Govt, has False Claim, does Misappropriation, false Warning and more.

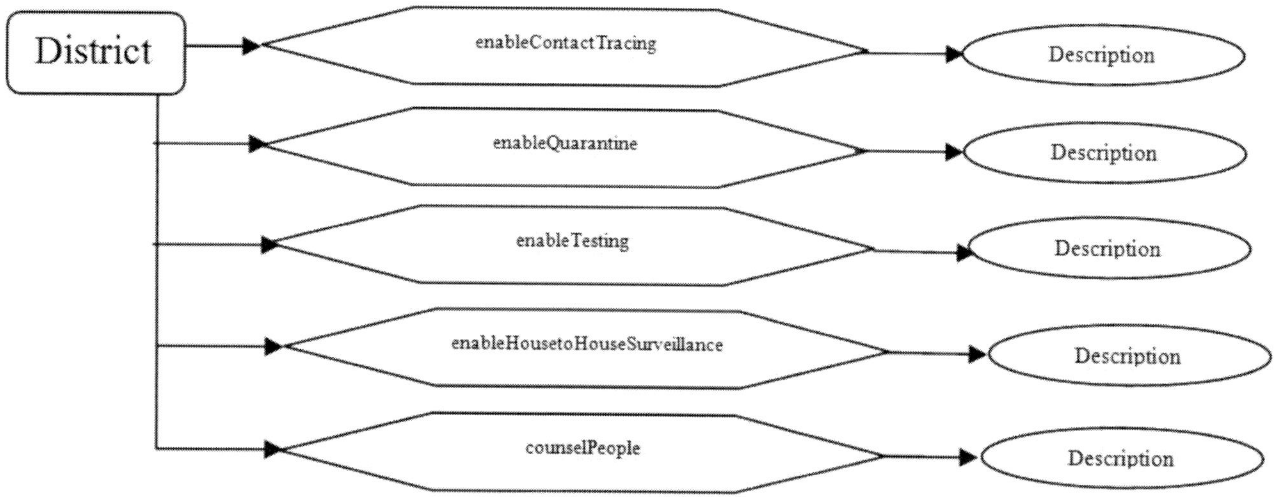

Figure 7a. Properties derived from containment policies.

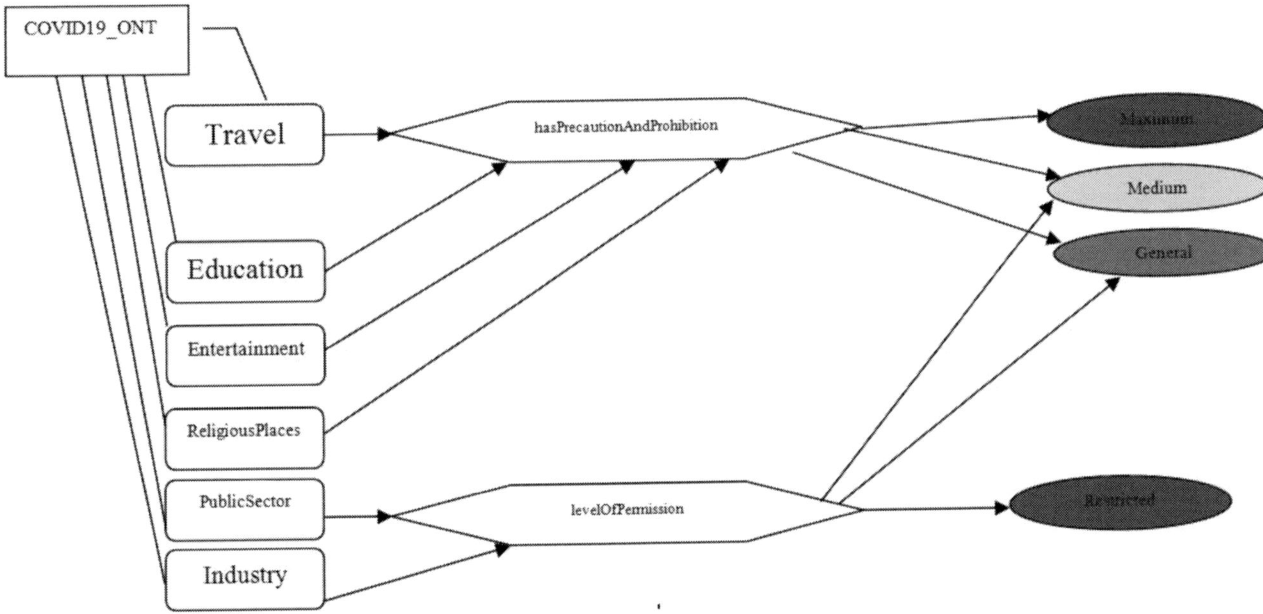

Figure 7b. Properties derived from various industries and sectors.

Once the properties are identified, the next job is the mapping of the policies to the semantic web rules. This task is furnished by the Policy To SWRule Mapper Agent. All the policies framed by the government are translated into a formal semantic web rule language called SWRL. These translated policies are then called rules. For simplicity, the legal polices converted into SWRL are enumerated below. The social, zonal and containment policies can be converted into SWRL by similar means [31].

1. Person(?p) ^ obstructsGovt()->Section51(?p)
2. Person(?p)^hasFalseClaim()->Section52(?p)
3. Person(?p)^doesMisappropriation()->Section53(?p)
4. Person(?p)^givesFalseWarning()->Section54(?p)
5. GovtEmployee(?g)^commitsOffence()->Section55(?g)
6. GovtEmployee(?g)^hasFailureInDuty()->Section56(?g)
7. Person(?p)^hasContradictionOfOrder->Section57(?p)
8. Company(?c)^commitsOffence()->Section58(?c)
9. GovtEmployee(?g)^hasPrevSectionForProsecution()->Section59(?g)
10. Person(?p)^disobeysPromulgatedOrder->Section188IPC(?p)

The above line means that if there is a person p and he obstructs government then he becomes the member of Section 51 class. The remaining SWRL rules can be understood in the same manner.

Reasoner Agent

The function of the Reasoner Agent is to perform the inference mechanism exploiting the Drools reasoner through the OWLAPI. The OWLAPI code used to create SWRL rule for obstructs Govt is shown in the excerpt below. The remaining rules can be added using similar code. After the inference mechanism takes place, all the SWRL rules get executed and the ontology may enter in another state with individual objects being made instances of another classes and fresh property assignment. Like, in our example if a person 'obstructs Govt' then it made the instance of Section 51 Class. Another worthy example of inferencing is Zone allotment into Red, Orange and Green on the basis of Corona cases. This can be shown in Figure 9. According to the magnitude of the cases, doubling rate and travel history the districts become the member of respective zone classes. And when the attributes of the cases change then these districts are reassigned membership of the new zone class.

As any district is assigned a zone, then that zone specific guidelines and rulings in terms of government policies are endorsed over the district. In our designed MAS, these zonal guidelines and rulings are bound with the Red, Orange and Green zone classes. So, as soon as a district becomes a member of any zone, the respective policies are enacted by the MAS. If a district changes its zone, the new policies are enforced according to the new zonal guideline and rulings.

So, the whole process of zone allotment and policies enactment is conducted by the MAS with minimum human intervention.

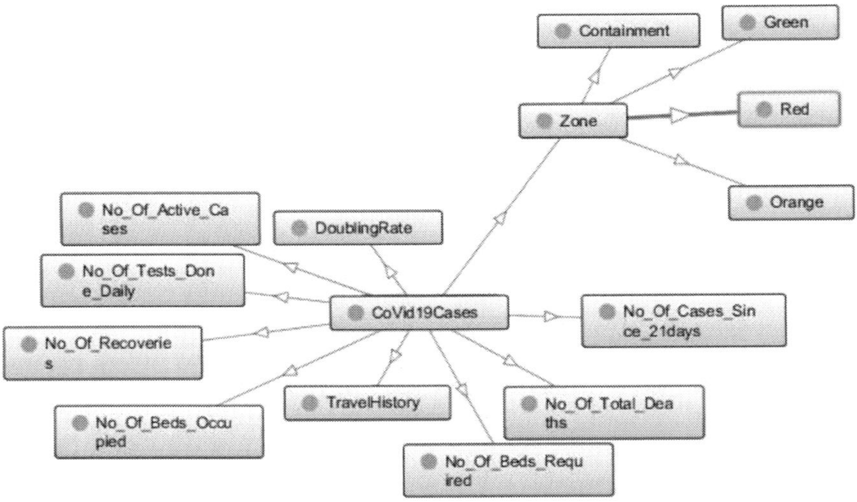

Figure 8. Zone allotments on the basis of COVID-19 Cases.

Conclusion and Future Scope

The authors have presented this chapter with deep analysis of the current pandemic situation worldwide. The design consists of a multi-agent system supported by a thorough knowledgebase, Covid19_ONT, developed and enriched in Protégé 5.2.0. NLP is used to extract the information regarding COVID-19 from valuable sources like mygov.in, who.int, nhs.uk and others. The authors have used JAPE and Gazetteer from GATE java package. Protégé 5.2.0 and its tools, OntoGraph, OWLviz and Drools reasoner are used along with OWLAPI and SWRLAPI to query and infer the COVID19_ONT ontology. The MAS is capable to randomly assign zones to any district according to the values of the attributes of COVID-19 cases. The MAS also provides guidelines and rulings under government policies for each district.

As future scope, this system can be improvised by advanced measures of knowledge extraction incorporating less time so that the process of knowledge extraction and ontology population may be streamlined.

References

[1] Singhal, Tanu. "A review of coronavirus disease-2019 (COVID-19)." *The Indian Journal of Pediatrics* (2020): 1-6.

[2] Roy, Deblina, et al. "Study of knowledge, attitude, anxiety & perceived mental healthcare need in Indian population during COVID-19 pandemic." *Asian Journal of Psychiatry* (2020): 102083.

[3] Young, Tom, et al. "Recent trends in deep learning based natural language processing." *IEEE Computational intelligence magazine* 13.3 (2018): 55-75.

[4] Otter, Daniel W., Julian R. Medina, and Jugal K. Kalita. "A survey of the usages of deep learning for natural language processing."

IEEE Transactions on Neural Networks and Learning Systems (2020).

[5] Chen, Long, et al. "Extracting medications and associated adverse drug events using a natural language processing system combining knowledge base and deep learning." *Journal of the American Medical Informatics Association* 27.1 (2020): 56-64.

[6] Reitemeyer, Benedikt, and Hans-Georg Fill. "Ontology-Driven Enterprise Modeling: A Plugin for the Protégé Platform." *Enterprise, Business-Process and Information Systems Modeling*. Springer, Cham, 2019. 212-226.

[7] Ding, Yuxin, Rui Wu, and Xiao Zhang. "Ontology-based knowledge representation for malware individuals and families." *Computers & Security* 87 (2019): 101574.

[8] Moape, Tebatso G., Sunday O. Ojo, and Etienne A. van Wyk. "A framework for appropriate pedagogical use of conceptual metaphor in computing." *2017 International Conference on Computing Networking and Informatics (ICCNI)*. IEEE, 2017.

[9] Ordóñez, Armando, et al. "Comparing drools and ontology reasoning approaches for automated monitoring in telecommunication processes." *Procedia Computer Science* 95 (2016): 353-360.

[10] Thu, Ei Ei, and Nwe Nwe. "Model driven development of mobile applications using drools knowledge-based rule." *2017 IEEE 15th International Conference on Software Engineering Research, Management and Applications (SERA)*. IEEE, 2017.

[11] Deyab, Rodwan Bakkar. *Ontology-based information extraction from learning management systems*. MS thesis. Universidade de Évora, 2017.

[12] Webster, Kellie. *Improved Coreference Resolution Using Cognitive Insights* (2016).

[13] Shankhdhar, Gaurav Kant, and Manuj Darbari. "Introducing Two Level Verification Model for Reduction of Uncertainty of Message Exchange in Inter Agent Communication in Organizational-Multi-Agent Systems Engineering, O-MaSE." *IOSR Journal of Computer*

Engineering (IOSR-JCE) IOSR Journal of Computer Engineering (IOSR-JCE) 19 (2017): 08-18.

[14] Shankhdhar, Gaurav Kant, et al. "Fuzzy Approach to Select Most Suitable Conflict Resolution Strategy in Multi-Agent System." *2019 International Conference on Cutting-edge Technologies in Engineering (ICon-CuTE)*. IEEE, 2019.

[15] Mishra, Sumit Kumar, and V. K. Singh. "Building Semantic Information Retrieval System for Legal Cases From Heterogeneous Adapted and Diverse Data Sources Using Extended GAIA Methodology for Multi Agent System." *2018 3rd International Conference On Internet of Things: Smart Innovation and Usages (IoT-SIU)*. IEEE, 2018.

[16] Kant, Gaurav, et al. "Legal Semantic Web-A Recommendation System." *International Journal of Applied Information Systems (IJAIS)* 7 (2014).

[17] Shankhdhar, Gaurav Kant, and Manuj Darbari. "Building custom, adaptive and heterogeneous multi-agent systems for semantic information retrieval using organizational-multi-agent systems engineering, O-MaSE." *2016 2nd International Conference on Advances in Computing, Communication, & Automation (ICACCA) (Fall)*. IEEE.

[18] Wang, Cuiyan, et al. "Immediate psychological responses and associated factors during the initial stage of the 2019 coronavirus disease (COVID-19) epidemic among the general population in China." *International journal of environmental research and public health* 17.5 (2020): 1729.

[19] Sahu, Kamal Kant, et al. "India Fights Back: COVID-19 Pandemic." *Heart & Lung: The Journal of Cardiopulmonary and Acute Care* (2020).

[20] Agoramoorthy, Govindasamy. "India fights hard to neutralize the spread of COVID-19." *Infection Control & Hospital Epidemiology* (2020): 1-1.

[21] Sharma, Suresh Kumar, et al. "COVID-19: Guidance Outlines on Infection Prevention and Control for Health Care Workers." *Indian Journal of Community Health* 32.1 (2020): 9-16.

[22] Cunningham, Hamish, et al. *The GATE user guide* (2002).

[23] Kadar, Manuella, and Adrian Tulbure. "An automated knowledge discovery framework with multi-agent systems - KDMAS." *2017 International Conference on Engineering, Technology and Innovation (ICE/ITMC)*. IEEE, 2017.

[24] Chi, Nai-Wen, Yu-Huei Jin, and Shang-Hsien Hsieh. "Developing base domain ontology from a reference collection to aid information retrieval." *Automation in Construction* 100 (2019): 180-189.

[25] Qiu, Jianyin, et al. "A nationwide survey of psychological distress among Chinese people in the COVID-19 epidemic: implications and policy recommendations." *General psychiatry* 33.2 (2020).

[26] Holmes, Emily A., et al. "Multidisciplinary research priorities for the COVID-19 pandemic: a call for action for mental health science." *The Lancet Psychiatry* (2020).

[27] Shetti, Nagaraj P., et al. "Invasion of novel corona virus (COVID-19) in Indian territory." *Sensors International* (2020): 100012.

[28] Sharma, Surbhi, et al. "Current treatment protocol for COVID-19 in India." *Sensors International* (2020): 100013.

[29] Nomani, M. Z. M., et al. "Quarantine Law Enforcement & Corona Virus (COVID-19) Pandemic in India." *Journal of X'idian University* 14.4 (2020): 536-542.

[30] Singh, Shashikant. "Analyasis of Disaster Management under the Lens of Legal Aspect of India with Special References to COVID-19." *Tathapi with ISSN 2320-0693 is an UGC CARE Journal* 19.20 (2020): 157-176.

[31] G. K. Shankhdhar, M. Darbari, "Implementation of Validation of Requirements in Agent Development by means of Ontology," *IJCESE Online*, 6(7):1129-1135.

[32] Horridge, Matthew, and Sean Bechhofer. "The owl api: A java api for owl ontologies." *Semantic web* 2.1 (2011): 11-21.

[33] Horridge, Matthew, and Sean Bechhofer. "The OWL API: a Java API for working with OWL 2 ontologies." *Proceedings of the 6th International Conference on OWL: Experiences and Directions-Volume 529*. CEUR-WS.org, 2009.

[34] O'Connor, Martin J., et al. "The SWRLAPI: A Development Environment for Working with SWRL Rules." *OWLED*. 2008.

[35] O'Connor, M. J., et al. "The SWRLAPI: A Development Environment for Working with SWRL Rules. OWL: Experiences and Directions." *5th International Workshop, Karlsruhe, Germany*. 2008.

In: Intelligent Information Retrieval … ISBN: 978-1-68507-301-5
Editors: Parma Nand et al. © 2021 Nova Science Publishers, Inc.

Chapter 3

AN OVERVIEW OF ONTOLOGY-BASED ARTIFICIAL INTELLIGENCE SERVICES IN HEALTH CARE SYSTEMS

R. S. M. Lakshmi Patibandla[1,*], B. Tarakeswara Rao[2], V. Lakshman Narayana[3] and V. Sesha Srinivas[4]

[1]Vignan's Foundation for Science, Technology, and Research, Andhra Pradesh, India

[2]Kallam Haranadhareddy Institute of Technology, Guntur, AP, India

[3]Vignan's Nirula Institute of Technology & Science for Women, Andhra Pradesh, India

[4]RVR&JC CE, College of Engineering Guntur, India

ABSTRACT

Service Computing includes an interdisciplinary focal point that coordinates science and age to connect the space between big business administrations and mastery Technology (IT) contributions. The inescapable idea of contributions figuring control is shown in the greatest venture settings. In way of life, new business administration developments will create an eminent, insights economy to least difficult

* Corresponding Author's E-mail: patibandla.lakshmi@gmail.com.

eat up steam as every purchaser and business utilization of the Internet of Things (IoT) innovations are progressed. Inside and out, we are drawing nearer to a period of Artificially Intelligent (AI) contributions, which are conveyed in multi-scale, complex assigned models. These AI administrations are routinely designed from significant level computational knowledge that uses rising investigative strategies identified with Big Data, Web analysis, information and text mining, Artificial Intelligence, semantic web, and a lot of different advances. At a methodological and innovative difficulties. For the duration of this chapter, service computing, the necessity for service computing, capabilities and applications of carrier computing, security and privateness issues, and Trust associated problems in fitness care services are certainly represented. Equivalent time, it'll become progressively fundamental to compute specialized and reasonable difficulties and to recognize decent practices learned through understanding. The arranging, improvement, and arrangement of ML contributions blessing novel.

Keywords: services, ontology, healthcare, AI, computing

INTRODUCTION

Services computing control involves: Ensuring administrations figuring approach is aligned with how the business oversees IT and how it's lined up with a hierarchical methodology, planning, fabricating, sourcing, and sending processing answers which may be flexible, trusted, effective, and adapt to Quality of Service desires, and Supervision all issues related with corporate and IT contributions tasks and assets each all through big business areas and inside spaces like account and healthcare. Also, analysts, organizations, and policymakers have seized on Machine Learning (ML) contributions to help their choices (Togias et al., 2010). ML administrations will catalyze keen utility zones like automatons and mechanical figuring. ML administrations will, in any case, improve with investigation discipline upgrades in locales like measurements/text mining, prescient examination, and calculations that model inordinate degree reflections in records through the utilization of several preparing layers with complex structures or non-straight changes (Usip et al., 2017). AI as a carrier, the idea of the whole thing as a provider refers to any software program with a purpose to be referred to as upon throughout a network because it uses cloud computing. In most cases, the software program is available off the shelf, which means that you honestly can buy it from a third-party vendor, make a couple of tweaks, and begin the use of it nearly immediately, albeit it hasn't been customized to your machine (Jain, S. et al., 2017).

For organizations that can't or are unwilling to create their very own clouds and construct, test, and utilize their personal AI structures, AI-as-a carrier is that the solution. Like different areas a carrier options, an equivalent technique is implemented to artificial intelligence: Allowing the corporate to specialize in their core commercial enterprise, now not becoming data and system getting to know experts, keeping costs transparent, considerably lowering the threat of investment, Increasing the blessings from records, increasing strategic flexibility, because AIas-a-carrier is bendy and dynamic (Julien Bidot et al., 2011). If we apprehend AIaaS as AI off the shelf, what are we getting as soon as we purchase a carrier? The following are the Well-recognized kinds of AIaaS encompass: Bots and digital assistance (Simons, S. et al., 2017). These can include, for example, chatbots that use Natural Language Processing (NLP) algorithms to discover from a verbal exchange with the citizenry and imitate the language patterns whilst presenting answers. This frees up customer support personnel to specialize in extra complex responsibilities (Jain, V. et al., 2016). These are the foremost extensively used sort of AIaaS immediately.

Cognitive computing APIs, short for software programming interface, APIs are how for builders to feature a particular generation or service into the appliance they may be built without writing the code from scratch (Sattar et al., 2021). Common alternatives for APIs include NLP, laptop speech and computer imagination and prescient, translation, understanding mapping, search, and emotion detection. Machine learning frameworks are tools that developers can use to create their model that learns over time from existing company information. Machine learning knowledge is typically related to massive data but can produce other uses and these frameworks offer a way to create in the system getting to know obligations without having the massive records environment (Despres S. et al., 2018). Fully-managed gadget mastering services, if device gaining knowledge of frameworks are the number one step closer to system studying, this selection may be a way to upload in the richer system getting to know abilities the usage of templates, prebuilt fashions, and drag-and-drop tools to help builders in constructing a more custom-designed device studying framework.

APPLICATIONS OF AI SERVICES

AI in Healthcare is the greatest vital wagers are on upgrading influenced individual results and lessening charges. Organizations are applying gadgets to figure out how to shape higher and snappier judgments than people. One of the charming respected human services innovations is IBM Watson. It gets tongue and may likewise respond to questions mentioned of it. The gadget mines influenced individual information and others to be had records causes near make a theory, which was at the time manages with a conviction attaining blueprint. Further AI programs unite exploiting on the web simulated well-being partners and chatbots to aid sufferers and social insurance customers find clinical data, timetable arrangements, catch the charging technique, and complete distinctive managerial strategies (Bouhissi et al., 2019). A variety of AI innovations is furthermore becoming accustomed to are anticipating, battle, and capture pandemics like COVID-19.

AI in Business, Machine acing calculations are being remembered for examination and purchaser relationship the executives (CRM) frameworks to reveal realities on the way to higher serve customers. Chatbots are incorporated keen on spots to flexibly instant suppliers on the way to customers (Bonini et al., 2021). Automation of procedure spots ingests moreover turn into a point amid examiners in the field of education and the field of information technology.

AI in Education, AI can robotize estimating, generous teachers longer. In this analysis undergrads then modify to their desires, supporting the works of art at their one-of-a-kind pace. Computer-based intelligence coaches can offer extra help to understudies, guaranteeing they stay music. What's more, it can exchange wherein and how understudies learn, perhaps usurping an insufficient instructor (Yadav U et al., 2018).

AI in Finance, Computer-based intelligence in nearby to household money programs, as Intuit Mint or TurboTax, is disquieting fiscal formations. Solicitations like these collect non-open measurements and flexible currency allied supervision. Dissimilar tasks, as IBM Watson, are done to the strategy for acquiring for a household. At present, AI user interface design plays out a mess of switching on Wall Street (Narula, G. S. et al., 2018).

AI in Law, the development method - choosing over records - in law is frequently intense for societies. Utilizing AI to help mechanize the lawful venture's work escalated procedures are sparing time and improving customer administration. Law enterprises are the utilization of framework figuring out how to clarify realities and anticipate impacts, PC vision to order, and concentrate insights from documents and tongue preparing to decipher demands for records (Patel, A et al., 2020).

AI in Manufacturing, Manufacturing has been present at the main edge of joining robots addicted to the exertion practice (Jain, Sarika et al., 2019). For example, a monetary robot that had been at basically any event customized on the way to complete distinct tasks and insulated as of social laborers, ever more capacity as per cobots: Smaller, concert numerous task machines that squad up by way of individuals then battle obligation used for more noteworthy parts of the canvases in dispersal centers, production line flooring, and different workspaces (Petnga, et al., 2016).

AI in banking, Banks are effectively utilizing chatbots to shape their clients mindful of contributions and contributions and to deal with exchanges that do no longer require human intercession. Simulated intelligence advanced aides are becoming accustomed to upgrade and cut the costs of consistency with banking guidelines. Banking organizations additionally are the utilization of AI to improve their dynamic for advances and to line financial assessment restrictions and recognize subsidizing openings (Titi S. et al., 2020).

AI in transportation, Additionally, to AI's basic situation in working self-ruling vehicles, AI innovation is used in transportation to oversee traffic, expect flight deferrals, and make sea dispatching more secure and more prominent effective (Mishra Tiwari et al., 2020).

NEED AND CHALLENGES OF AI SERVICES

The approvals of deploying AIaaS have heaps in not unusual with the overall blessings of some primarily consumed based (i.e., on-demand) software service. For instance, unified scalability can be a significant factor because it allows companies to start small and gradually scale up their AI operations over time (in step with project-specific requirements) (Titi et al., 2019). In the course of a scene wherein the necessity for super-speedy graphical consumer interfaces. As the cost of (GPUs) as well as parallel machines increases, AIaaS comes in handy because it helps IT managers to incorporate and use the most up-to-date AI-powered infrastructure without having to worry about the high costs. Since AIas-a-Service can overcome the challenges faced by the comparatively complex design of traditional AI solutions, it is referred to as AIas-a-Service. But there's one more benefit to those off-the-shelf AI solutions: total accountability. Ours is a data-driven world, and the value of real-time decision-making skills cannot be overstated (Jain, Sarika et al., 2021). This is a driving force behind AIaaS responses.

The amount of data collected by specialized smart sensors, UAVs, and various types of IoT programs is growing at an exponential pace, necessitating enhanced, intelligent statistics management, use, accessibility, and safety. AIaaS is suitable for more intelligent big data management as well as assisting computer systems in performing complex tasks (Lai et al., 2020). The development/deployment time is reduced since these offerings are available from suppliers as ready-to-use kits. The fact that AIaaS is used by almost everyone (thanks to the user-friendly underlying algorithms) contributes to its success. The increasing demand for faster GUIs and customized APIs are driving this sector. AIaaS can have massive competitive advantages for cloud providers but businesses in general.

Challenges in AI Services

Rather than charge exorbitant amounts with high overheads, consumers should pay based on how much they use the services (Hu, X. et al., 2020). The key to AIaaS is to make money for businesses by implementing smarter AI-powered projects with lower operating costs. Although it has several benefits including easy usability, AIaaS (like every other modern technology carrier!) has some downside. Users who use third-party AI tools for data, effects, or statistics can encounter unexpected delays (Rocha, B. D. et al., 2020). Since a lot of enterprise-critical data has to be exchanged with third parties, the increased dependence on third-party service providers can lead to data protection concerns. Since a significant volume of enterprise-critical data has to be exchanged with third-party vendors. The key here is to make sure that the AIaaS you choose has good protection and data governance requirements in place to avoid unauthorized access. Once we get past the initial cost-benefits of AIaaS (over conventional AI), the probability of fees rising in the long run as the generation becomes more nuanced and complex becomes evident. Since AIaaS is sold as a kit, it is impossible to identify the internal AI mechanisms even though the information inputs and expected outcomes are known (Reyes-Pena et al., 2019). As a result, the AI offerings' overall openness is diminished. Over the next few quarters, the generation will advance, and that we can fairly conclude that virtually all of these difficult circumstances will be satisfactorily resolved.

Communication Framework for the AI Services

In Artificial Intelligence (AI), the old-style arranging issue incorporates a gathering of administrators, one fundamental nation, and one-point country. The occasion of an administrator is known as a strategic. A nation can be an immovable of great centers (i.e., started up predicates). A planet public can advance; for instance, it variations while a mission is practiced because of the way that each done strategically by and large an impact on the predominant worldwide realm (Jain, S. et al., 2018). The objective is too excellent and arranges assignments in a phase that license to accomplish the point nation as of the primer nation. Errands are oftentimes finished for the length of a universal nation; since certain preconditions keep up all through this state. Each undertaking is identified with preconditions and impacts.

An idea comprises obligations and worldly and causal connections amongst them. Prescribed Structure, the PA typifies a request motor for AI arranging (Jain, S. et al., 2020). This program depends on a legitimate structure that coordinates Partial-Order Causal-Link (POCL) arranging and Hierarchical Task Network (HTN) making arrangements. This half and half arranging system utilizes an ADL-like illustration of situations and crucial activities (crude obligations). Shapes, prerequisites, and impacts of duties are determined through methods of a part of the first-request rationale (Mishra Tiwari et al., 2020). Dynamic obligations are normally sensitive by so-known as deterioration techniques, which give task systems (fractional plans) that depict how the comparing strategy is regularly understood. Fractional plans may likewise contain rundown and crude obligations. With that, chains of the importance of commitments and related methodologies are consistently wont to encode different approaches to achieve a theoretical task.

Arrangement expects that during stylish a mapping can be characterized as fourfold. More or less, our arrangement utilizes a blend of phrased approaches, which endeavor to string similitude among names of ontologies by auxiliary methodologies, which trust on the state of the ontologies (Peng et al., 2019).

For evaluating the term comparability of standards and assets, we utilize the Levenshtein alter separation metric among two strings, progressively alluring with an equivalents database that we keep up (an outer helpful asset along with WordNet could likewise be utilized). In any case, the lexical closeness isn't continually alright to check that guidelines are semantically good. We, along these lines, examine whether their immediate predecessors and relatives notwithstanding kin substances rate a lexical similitude (Mishra Tiwari et al., 2019). Thusly, we can decide the auxiliary significance of guidelines. The strategy for the arrangement has its confinements. Good results are procured when the info ontologies are inside the equivalent region and besides no ordered connections (i.e., limitations) among standards are not considered. The yield of the arrangement strategy is an OWL philosophy that comprises OWL style comparability affirmations that transmit identical thoughts as of the information ontologies. A case of arrangement is demonstrated in Figure 2.

Thinking about the dynamic variety of the work processes, most presentation inconveniences fall inside the official of the contraptions to the rundown administrations (Govindaraj, Suganya et al., 2018). From tests finished in our IE testbed for the circumstance gave inside the start, a huge time of the work process introduction is credited to questioning the gadget's ontologies. The exhibition of the OM perspective is imperative, seeing that a huge weight of the dynamic variety is that the office of the first fitting gadget for a theoretical transporter, and when you consider that numerous coefficients must be taken underneath thought before choosing an instrument (area, customer, nearness, and so on).

In the wake of running the circumstance on various occasions, the ensuing outcomes had been created: (1) 80% of the ideal opportunity for work process statement is that the time wanted for the questions; (2) Questions have a start-up capacity that is straight to the measure of strategies that occur esoteric the extreme cluster; (3) The usual time of work process introduction is direct to the measure of contributions may get a kick out of the chance to tie.

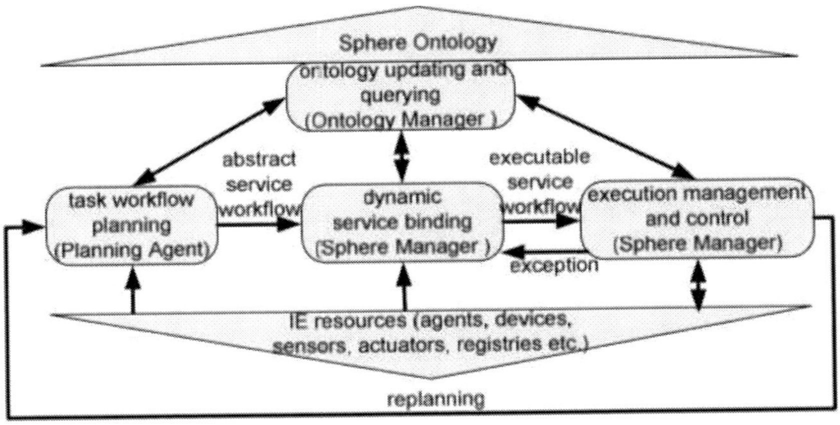

Figure 1.

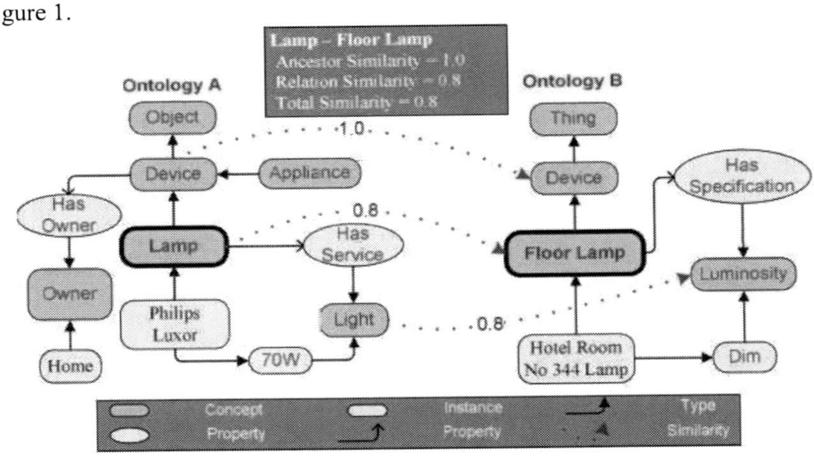

Figure 2.

Ontology Services in Health Care

Ontology Services in Health Care Ontologies in measurements science have their sources in manmade consciousness wherein the absence of a typical comprehension of a site of pastime introduced a decent estimated boundary to developing and sharing collected skill bases, and thusly to fabricate interoperable structures. Ontologies are a deliberation of the real world; they depict the ideas identified with a site or relic and through an efficient distinct framework feature the requirements of those norms (Saat, Nur et al., 2016). The utilization of ontologies in biomedical informatics is pleasantly settled, anyway, in the general execution estimation field the strategy is early; hence sharing and participating to build regular ontologies is a basic segment of emerging this zone. Mutually their grammatical and semantic structures, ontologies grant for proper classification and calculation of the connections amongst things existence depicted. As a result of utilizing a derivation motor, the affirmed connections between things might be figured.

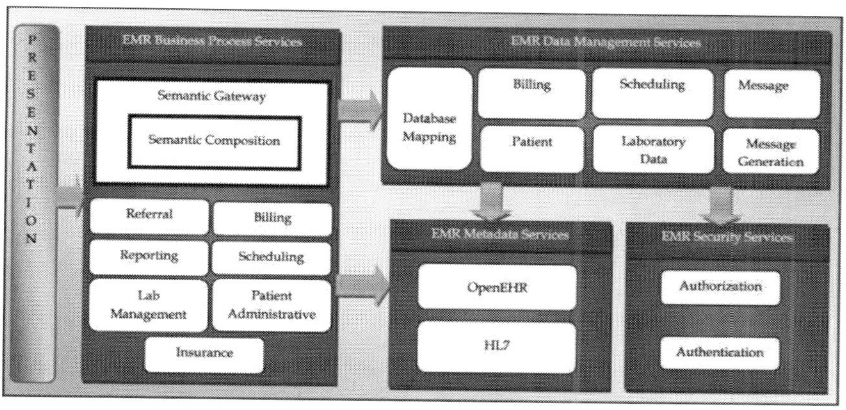

Figure 3.

Any infringement of sayings and rationale imperatives will be recognized. The measured methodology characteristic in ontologies (accomplished using a not irregular jargon of authentic expressions and unequivocal revelatory skill) way cosmology is extendable to be utilized with various related ontologies. Besides, ontological styles are consistently calculable importance it is practical to reason new records dependent on the basic variant. Whereas ontologies are normal in biomedicine and are more and more utilized in planning oversaw expressions and allusion phrasings, there are slight examinations addicted to utilizing ontologies completed to wellness realities structures themselves, or in help of social insurance execution estimation. Short of mutual or normalized lexical and semantic replicas, trustworthy and exact difference of execution all through segments and geographical fringes is unfeasible. At this point investigate the product of an ontological model structured mutually to abstract then quantify electric wellbeing realities change among wellbeing elements in an enormous neighborhood human services contraption in Ontario, Canada, and to check the unwavering quality of the gathered records.

Table 1. Categories of Healthiness object in a regional healthcare system

Entity Type: Health	**Subclasses**
Entities in the Hospital Industry	Health Services, Learning, Community, Small, Variable Continuous Care/Healing (5)
Entities involved in primary care	Healthcare Services Model, Campus Health Services, Treatment Center, Government Service, Solo Practice, Group Practice, Family Health Group, Family Health Team, Family Health Network
Physician Specialty Organizations	Single Practice, Group Practice
Entities that offer diagnostic facilities	Laboratory, Imaging
Entities that offer residential care	Long Term Care, Nursing Home, Palliative Care
Entities that provide community-based health services	Counseling, mental health clinics, pharmacies, sports medicine clinics, and treatment services are also available in the community.
Entities of Community Care Access Centers	Community Care Access Centres
Entities that are part of the public health system	Public Health Unit
Entities that provide emergency medical services	Entity for Medical Services

Security and Privacy Issues in Health Care

AI in social insurance has obvious rapid advancements in the course of the most recent couple of years. The most widely recognized AI application today, gadgets becoming more acquainted with, can engage care merchants to shape higher analyses, offer better patient consideration, and improve get section to medicinal services. So also, their wonderful capacity for AI to develop the territories of human services security and assurance. Whenever utilized appropriately, AI can change medicinal services' privateness and security. Whenever abused, it might cause a moral breakdown and heap legitimate issues. During this whitepaper, discover how AI can offer additional help for human services privateness and security, including the preferences previously acknowledged using AI in medicinal services. What cares merchants and privateness and security experts ought to limit considerations concerning the ethical utilization of AI to downsize lawful, consistent, and administrative hazards. Three rules that associations can use to control their inclination of age and merchants. Round out the shape at the best possible to get your duplicate of this manual to the most cutting-edge advancements and worries in the social insurance AI age.

CONCLUSION

This research closes with a summary of Ontology-Based AI Services in Health Care Systems. This portrays the need and difficulties of AI administrations; the work process the executive's frameworks have not been utilized for dynamic conditions requiring programmed versatile conduct. The work process depicts the relationship among contributions and if a specialist is spoken to through the kind of bearer, at that point the relationship among the merchants would be reasonable to indicate. Inside the not-so-distant future, the synchronous arrangement of various work processes in the indistinguishable space, which can intention synchronization issues wherein particular work processes may likewise vie for equivalent resources and perform clashing activities.

REFERENCES

Bonini J. A., Da Silva M. D., Pereira R., Mozzaquatro B. A., Martini R. G., Librelotto G. R. (2021) An Application of Ontological Engineering for Design and Specification of Ontocancro. In: Panuccio G., Rocha M., Fdez-Riverola F., Mohamad M., Casado-Vara R. (eds) *Practical Applications of Computational Biology & Bioinformatics, 14th International Conference (PACBB 2020). PACBB 2020. Advances in Intelligent Systems and Computing*, vol 1240. Springer, Cham. https:// doi.org/10.1007/978-3-030-54568-0_14.

Bouhissi, H. E., Salem, A. B. M., & Tari, A. (2019). Semantic enrichment of web services using linked open data. *International Journal of Web Engineering and Technology*, 14(4), 383-416.

Desprès, S. (2018). "oogo: Ontologie des Outils utiles à la Gestion d'Ontologies" [oogo: Ontology Tools useful for Ontology Management] In: *29es Journées Francophones d'Ingénierie des Connaissances* [*29th Francophone Knowledge Engineering Days*], IC 2018 163-178.

Govindaraj, Suganya & Dr. R. Porkodi (2018). *Ontology Based Information Extraction-A Review.*

Hu, X., & Liu, J. (2020). Ontology construction and evaluation of UAV FCMS software requirement elicitation considering geographic environment factors. *IEEE Access*, 8, 106165-106182.

Jain, S., & Meyer, V. (2018). Evaluation and refinement of emergency situation ontology. *International Journal of Information and Education Technology*, 8(10), 713-719.

Jain, Sarika & Patel, Archana (2019). *Smart Ontology-Based Event Identification*. 135-142. 10.1109/MCSoC.2019.00027.

Jain, S., Sharma, S., Natterbrede, J. M., & Hamada, M. (2020). Rule-Based Actionable Intelligence for Disaster Situation Management. *International Journal of Knowledge and Systems Science (IJKSS)*, 11(3), 17-32.

Jain, S., Shao, G., and Shin, S. J. (2017). Manufacturing data analytics using a virtual factory representation. *International Journal of Production Research*, 55(18):5450-5464.

Jain, S. (2018). Conceptualization of Indian Biodiversity by Using Semantic Web Technologies. In: *International Conference On Computational Vision and Bio Inspired Computing* (pp. 1445-1453). Springer, Cham.

Jain, Sarika, and Archana Patel (2021). "Semantic Contextual Reasoning to Provide Human Behavior." *arXiv preprint arXiv:2103.10694*.

Jain, V. I. S. H. A. L., & Prasad, S. V. A. V. (2016). Evaluation and Validation of ontology using Protégé Tool. *International Journal of Research in Engineering & Technology (IMPACT: IJRET) ISSN (E)*, 2321-8843.

Julien Bidot et al. (2011), Using AI Planning and Late Binding for Managing Service Workflows in Intelligent Environments, *IEEE Conference on Pervasive Computing and Communications*. pp: 156-163.

Lai, Phung & Phan, Nhat Hai & Hu, Han & Badeti, Anuja & Newman, David & Dou, Dejing (2020). *Ontology-based Interpretable Machine Learning for Textual Data.*

Mishra Tiwari, Sanju & Abraham, Ajith (2020). Semantic assessment of smart healthcare ontology. *International Journal of Web Information Systems*. ahead-of-print. 10.1108/IJWIS-05-2020-0027.

Mishra Tiwari, Sanju & Jain, Sarika & Abraham, Ajith & Shandilya, Smita (2019). Secure Semantic Smart HealthCare (S3HC). *Journal of Web Engineering*. 17. 617-646. 10.13052/jwe1540-9589.1782.

Mishra Tiwari, Sanju & Abraham, Ajith (2020). Semantic assessment of smart healthcare ontology. *International Journal of Web Information Systems*. ahead-of-print. 10.1108/IJWIS-05-2020-0027.

Narula, G. S., Wason, R., Jain, V., & Baliyan, A. (2018). Ontology mapping and merging aspects in semantic web. *Int. Rob. Auto J.*, 4(1), 00087.

Peng, Cong & Goswami, Prashant (2019). Meaningful Integration of Data from Heterogeneous Health Services and Home Environment Based on Ontology. *Sensors*. 19. 1747. 10.3390/s19081747.

Patel, A., Sharma, A., & Jain, S. (2020). An intelligent resource manager over terrorism knowledge base. *Recent Advances in Computer Science and Communications* (Formerly: Recent Patents on Computer Science), 13(3), 394-405.

Petnga, Leonard & Austin, Mark (2016). An ontological framework for knowledge modelling and decision support in cyber-physical systems. *Advanced Engineering Informatics*. 30. 77. 10.1016/j.aei.2015.12.003.

Reyes-Pena, C., & Tovar-Vidal, M. (2019). Ontology: Components and Evaluation, a Review. *Research in Computing Science* 148, 257-265.

Rocha, B. D., Silva, L., Batista, T., Cavalcante, E., & Gomes, P. (2020). An Ontology-based Information Model for Multi-Domain Semantic Modeling and Analysis of Smart City Data. In: *Proceedings of the Brazilian Symposium on Multimedia and the Web* (pp. 73-80).

Saat, Nur & Mohd Noah, Shahrul Azman (2016). Rule-based Approach for Automatic Ontology Population of Agriculture Domain. *Information Technology Journal*. 15. 46-51. 10.3923/itj.2016.46.51.

Sattar, Abdul & Ahmad, Mohammad Nazir & Salwana, Ely & Mahmood, Ahmad Kamil (2021). An Improved Methodology for Collaborative Construction of Reusable, Localized, and Shareable Ontology. *IEEE Access*. 10.1109/ACCESS.2021.3054412. 17463-17484.

Simons, S., Ab´e, P., and Neser, S. (2017). Learning in the art fab - the fully automated industry 4.0 learning factory of the university of applied sciences Darmstadt. *Procedia Manufacturing*, 9:81-88.

Togias, Konstantinos & Kameas, Achilles (2010). Ontology-Based Representation of UPnP Devices and Services for Dynamic Context-Aware Ubiquitous Computing Applications. *2010 Third*

International Conference on Communication Theory, Reliability, and Quality of Service. 220-225. 10.1109/CTRQ.2010.44.

Titi S., Ben Elhadj H., Chaari Fourati L. (2020) A Fuzzy-Ontology Based Diabetes Monitoring System Using Internet of Things. In: Jmaiel M., Mokhtari M., Abdulrazak B., Aloulou H., Kallel S. (eds) The Impact of Digital Technologies on Public Health in Developed and Developing Countries. ICOST 2020. *Lecture Notes in Computer Science,* vol 12157. Springer, Cham. https://doi.org/10.1007/978-3-030-51517-1_25.

Titi, Sondes & Elhadj, Hadda & Fourati, Lamia (2019). *An ontology-based healthcare monitoring system in the Internet of Things*. 319-324. 10.1109/IWCMC.2019.8766510.

Usip, Patience & Umoren, Moses & Inyang, Udoinyang & Mfonobong, Maurice & Ntekop (2017). An Ontology-Based Temporal Scheduling and Complexity Reduction Model for Timetabling Knowledge Management. Advances in Science, *Technology and Engineering Systems Journal*. 2. 10.25046/aj0203197.

Yadav U., Murthy B. K., Narula G. S., Duhan N., Jain V. (2018) EasyOnto: A Collaborative Semiformal Ontology Development Platform. In: Panigrahi B., Hoda M., Sharma V., Goel S. (eds) *Nature Inspired Computing. Advances in Intelligent Systems and Computing*, vol 652. Springer, Singapore. https://doi.org/10.1007/978-981-10-6747-1_1.

In: Intelligent Information Retrieval … ISBN: 978-1-68507-301-5
Editors: Parma Nand et al. © 2021 Nova Science Publishers, Inc.

Chapter 4

DLCDI: A NOVEL DEEP LEARNING MECHANISM FOR CHRONIC DISEASES IDENTIFICATION

Pokkuluri Kiran Sree*, PhD and Usha Devi N.
Department of CSE, Shri Vishnu Engineering College for Women (A), Bhimavaram, Andhra Pradesh India
Department of CSE, University College of Engineering, JNTU-Kakinada, Kakinada, Andhra Pradesh, India

ABSTRACT

Chronic disease identification is pronounced as the most critical problem in Bioinformatics. We have identified cancer identification, heart disease, and diabetes as potential chronic diseases that can be addressed quickly with a novel deep learning mechanism augmented with cellular automata (C.A.). The framework of C.A. with CNN (Convolution Neural Network) is used to identify the protein-coding regions in genomic DNA. Identifying the protein-coding region and analyzing these can be helpful for predicting the three diseases in particular. The proposed classifier DLCDI (Deep Learning Chronic Disease Identification)has considered eight neighborhood cellular

* Corresponding Author's E-mail: drkiransree@gmail.com.

automata to represent the state space, and we have developed the corresponding complemented/non complemented rules for the prediction. This is the first method that identifies PCR, and then these chronic diseases as identifying PCR itself is a highly complex process. We have taken 10,16,189 datasets from U.S. Center for Disease Control and Prevention on chronic disease indicators for training and testing the desired classifier. The model accuracy in predicting PCR was reported as 88.9%. DLCDI was robust and adaptable with a prediction accuracy of 81.23% for cancer prediction, 85.78% for heart disease, and 89.36% for Diabetes II prediction. We have compared DLCDI with the existing literature, i.e., methods predicting PCR, Cancer, Heart Diseases, Diabetes-II, and results were found promising.

Keywords: disease finding, cellular automata, deep learning, CNN

INTRODUCTION

Disease identification is a vital real-time problem addressed by many researchers for years. In these diseases, chronic diseases are the most dangerous diseases humanity faces (Gavhane et al., 2018). Among the chronic diseases, we have identified three of them that was sounded very dangerous for the health of humans identified by the U.S. health department. The three identified diseases are cancer, heart attack, and diabetes.

We have thoroughly studied the features of these diseases and found some commonalities among them. This solution needed a common platform that could be used to identify these diseases. A feasibility study was conducted on what type of technique can be applied to solve this problem.

Deep Learning is productive when massive data is available for training, and these models have solved many complicated, dynamic real-time problems with higher accuracy with time (Holzinger 2016). Shankar et al., have identified CNN as a unique class of neural networks that processes known data with grid topology (Shankar et al., 2020). CNN has many applications, and it operates on a mathematical operator, which is called convolution. It uses many linear operators, represented in matrix form, and then extracts the features of the samples. We propose a distinctive architecture that processes DNA sequence, and operates directly on the characters, and uses simple pooling operations & convolutions, which is termed as CNN augmented with the cellular automata rules to identify these diseases. The main challenge in this research is mapping the disease characteristics to CNN (Boulent et al., 2019) and proceed to train /test the classifier. This chapter is organized in this format; section 2 depicts the literature survey of various DL models, different C.A. methods, the standard methods of predicting these diseases, and provides the need to select this classifier to address this problem.

LITERATURE SURVEY

Review of Various Deep Learning Models

A Neural network that operates in a feedforward fashion uses only the connections between the nodes in the forward direction are termed Deep Forwarddd NN. It consists of various hidden layers to process large datasets. In general, these will operate in this fashion. Deep learning permits computational models of various preparing layers to learn and speak to information with different degrees of deliberation, copying how the cerebrum sees and comprehends multimodal data along these lines, certainly catching unpredictable structures of large-scale data. Deep learning is a wealthy group of techniques incorporating neural systems, progressive probabilistic models, and an assortment of unaided and managed highlight learning calculations. The ongoing flood of enthusiasm for profound learning strategies is because of the way that they have been appeared to outflank past best in class systems in a few errands, just as the wealth of complex information from various sources (e.g., visual, sound, clinical, social, and sensor). We have reviewed multiple types of DL methods referred by Deng, Naz, Ravi, Sajja, which can address our problem(Deng and Yu 2013), (Naz and Ahuja 2020), (Ravi et al., 2017) (Sajja and Kalluri 2020).

Review of Various Cellular Automata

Xiao et al., have explored the use of C.A. in design grouping with certain esteemed information (Xiao et al., 2020). A genetic algorithm is used to implement Fuzzy Cellular Automata, which is a particular class of C.A. Sree et al., (Sree and Devi Nedunuri 2020) has proposed a hypothesis and utilization of C.A. for design arrangement. A genetic algorithm is used to develop the fuzzy MACA (Chicco 2017). The same authors have additionally proposed the mistake of rectifying the ability of cell automata dependent on collective memory. The ideal C.A. is advanced with the definition of a reenacted toughening program, which can be helpful in VLSI innovation. We have reviewed various types of C.A. referred by Wolfram that can be applied for this technique.

Table 1. Different forms of CA

SNO	Various forms of C.A.	Informal Meaning
1	Additive- C.A.	Each transition is defined with either XNOR or XOR or combination.
2	Synchronous- C.A.	All states will have the same rules applied.
3	Asynchronous -C.A.	Each state can have its own rule.
4	Non-Linear -C.A.	Transitions are defined with non-linear rules
5	Null Boundary- C.A.	Right and left, most cell values are assumed as zeros.
6	Periodic Boundary -C.A.	Right and left, most cells are connected.
7	Uniform -C.A.	Transition function is applied in a linear fashion to all the cells
8	Hybrid -Automata	Rules are framed based on various combinations.
9	Multiple-CA	Combination of Uniform and Non-Uniform CA
10	Multi-Level CA	Use of different transition functions at each level

A simple classification strategy of C.A. with XOR logic was provided in Figure 2, where 011 is the starting state and 000 is the final state, which is called a basin that has a common property.

After the literature survey on various DL methods and C.A. types, we understood that CNN, with an embedding layer augmented with eight neighborhood C.A., would be a better classifier to solve the problem.

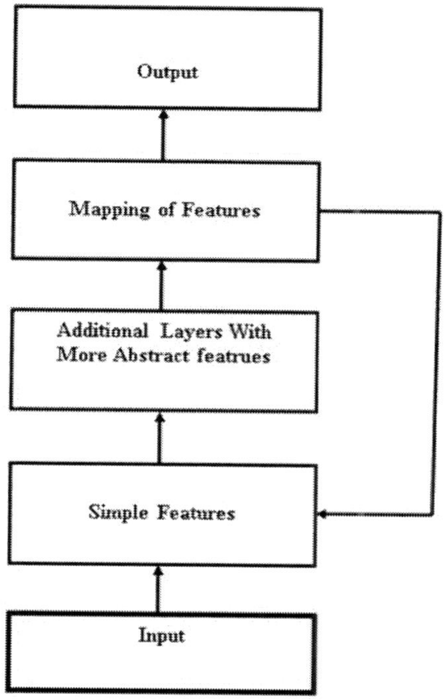

Figure 1. Learning with Deep Learning.

Review of Various Protein-Coding Region (PCR) Identification Systems

This section reports the pros and cons of several vital protein-coding region systems. The first one is a machine learning strategy that can learn from a set of examples. Many learning mechanisms are proposed with a Clonal algorithm, genetic algorithm, decision tree, and ILP (Inductive Logic Procedure). Machine learning can process different forms of data and will classify the data easily based on several rules (Schaefer et al., 2020).

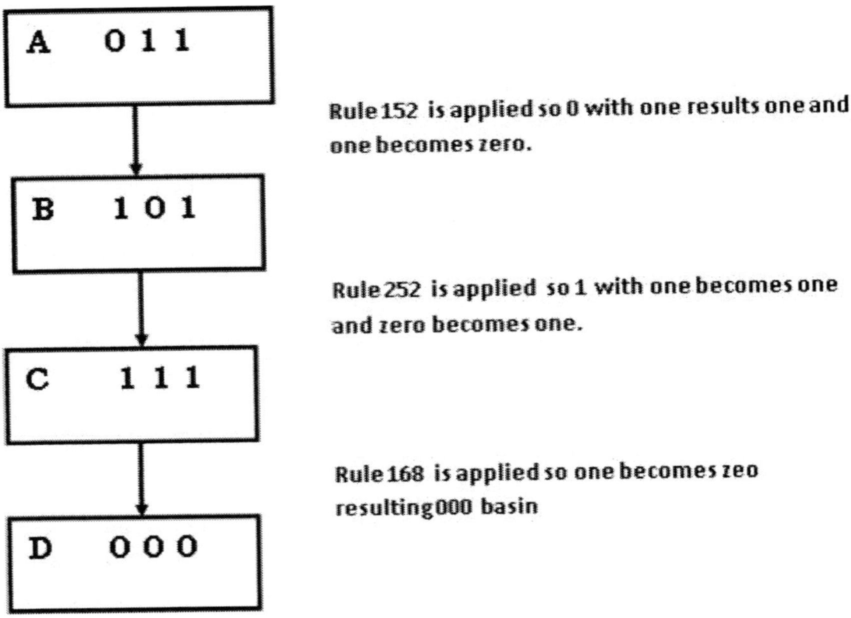

Figure 2. Example Classifier with XOR logic.

Decision Tree (DT)

Decision Tree performs decisions at various stages in a hierarchical order. Shouman, Salguero et al., have reviewed different decision trees in the context of pattern classifiers (Shouman, Turner, and Stocker 2011) (Soguero-Ruiz et al., 2020). Many decision trees are applied to this problem proposed by Yadel et al., (D. C. Yadav and Pal 2020), which are very significant CART, SPRINT, and C4.5.

Neural Networks (NN)

Many researchers have tried to address the problem of PCR using neural networks as these consist of several layers, with each one consisting of interconnecting nodes. Each node indeed produces a non-linear function of the received input. The network output is associated with a few nodes. Zhou et al., have (Zhou, Myrzashova, and Zheng 2020) proposed a feedback network, and the Hopfield network is used to predict PCR in a human genome.

Review of Various Heart Attack Prediction Systems

Heart disease or heart attack is pronounced as the deadliest one several patients have faced. The best heat disease predictor has to process large data sets, parameters and study the essential features for an accurate classifier (Martin-Isla et al., 2020). Many heart attack prediction systems are available. Still, there a room for a better classifier to predict the same. Alexander, C. An et al., has proposed a bigdata analytics method to identify the heart attack (Alexander and Wang 2017). This work was initially tested for a few patients and still needs to be improved. Shah et al., has studied the application of various data mining models to predict heart attack with few parameters considered (Shah, Patel, and Bharti 2020). S.S.Yadav et al., have studied the use of different feature selection methods (S. S. Yadav and Jadhav 2019) for better identification of heart attack and studied the effect of anxiety on the occurrence of the heart attack.

Review of Various Cancer Prediction Systems

Cruz et al., have studied multiple parameters to identify lung cancer using different data mining methods (Cruz and Wishart 2006). Authors have used many statistical classifiers with less precision calculation systems to predict caner with 65.7 probability. Al-Yasrij et al., have studied various conditions on which cancer patients can survive lifelong (Al-Yasriy et al., 2020). Daniel et al., have studied multiple parameters of sustainability and susceptibility of cancer patients(Danaee, Ghajini, and Hendrix 2017, Iqbal et al., studied various risk factors to be taken into account to predict cancer(Iqbal et al., 2021). We have reviewed different cancer prediction systems for developing a robust classifier (Krithiga and Geetha 2020), (Mostavi et al., 2020), (Xie et al. 2019).

Review of Different Diabetes Prediction Systems

Lai et al., have developed multiple techniques to prevent diabetes (Lai et al., 2019). Sneha et al., have studied various techniques and methods to overcome diabetes (Sneha and Gangil 2019). Zou et al., have surveyed what types of risk factors will reduce the risk of diabetes in the human body (Zou et al., 2018).

Summary of the Literature Survey

After an extensive literature survey, we understood that this problem needs a common platform to predict diseases. We found identifying the protein-coding region is the first step to detect these diseases. We also observed that identifying PCR will help to solve many problems other than the three diseases prediction also. We also infer that CNN augmented with C.A. can be a better classifier to predict PCR and then the related diseases.

Design of DLCDI

The data sets are collected from U.S. Center for Disease Control and Prevention from the CDV website. The design of DLCDI is shown in fig 3. We have obtained 5,02,968 data sets from the cited resource and processed these so that each will be collected in the form of three codons(words). After the preprocessing of these, hybrid C.A. rules are applied to the codons for initial computation.

These initially computed codons are processed by CNN, as shown in Figure 4. The codons (words) are given as input to the CNN, which will be passed to the embedding vector as these will cover come most of the traditional embedding problems.

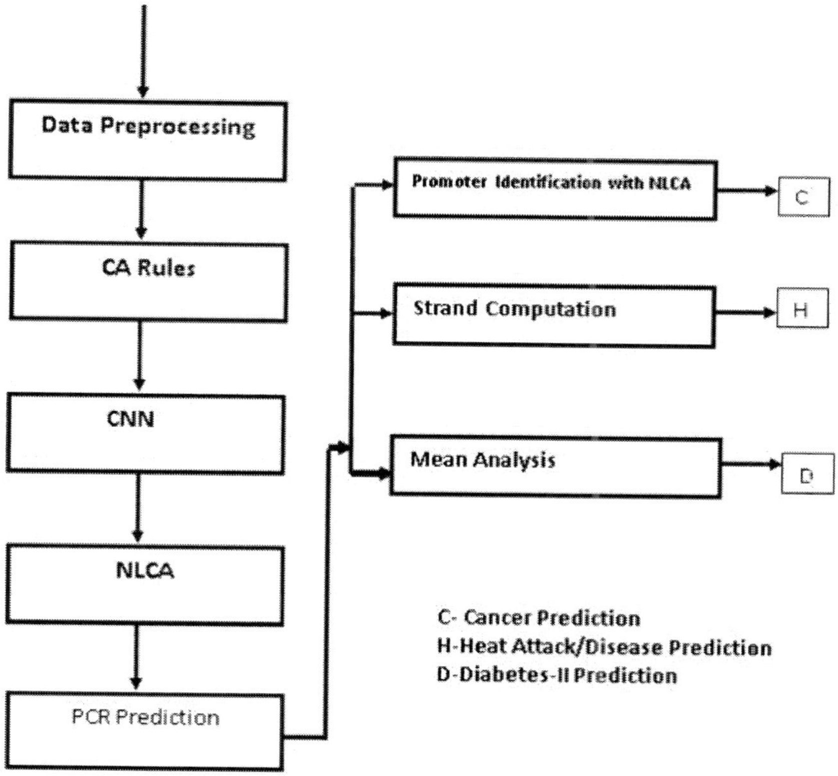

Figure 3. The Design of DLCDI.

We use a convolution mechanism to merge these functions to get a new process. Max polling reduces the size progressively, thus decreasing the calculation and the number of parameters. The last stage of CNN is termed the classification stage, where we have eight different classes to perform classification.

These eight classes are given input to a Non-Linear Cellular Automata algorithm, which operates as shown in Figure 5, to decide whether the sequence contains protein-coding is not. Once the series contains PCR, then we have to check whether this sequence includes any of these diseases (cancer, heart disease, and diabetes) or in combination. We perform promoter prediction using a C.A. classifier to predict whether this sequence contains cancer-causing attributes or not. We perform strand computing to predict whether the sequence contains any heart diseases or not. We perform a mean analysis method to predict whether this sequence contains diabetes or not.

Wolfram [8] has defined, the rule number can be the decimal number equivalent of the next state. In this context, when we consider three neighborhoods and two states for cellular automata, we can give 256 following different forms as in equations 1,2. Non Complemented rules are listed in Table 2.

$$\text{Complemented Rule 51}: q_i\overline{(t+1)} = q_i(t) \quad (1)$$

$$\text{Non Complemented 238}: q_i(t+1) = q_i(t) + q_{i+1}(\mathrm{t}) \quad (2)$$

Table 2. Rules without complementation

1	252	$q_{i-1} + q_{i+1} + q_i$
2	244	$q_{i} + q_{i-1}$
3	256	$q_{i-1} + q_i$
4	178	q_i
5	0	0

Let us consider the first state in Figure 5. The input is 0.2,.4,.6. The rules at the first stat say it has to depend on the right neighbor, so the transition state is 0.6,0.8,0.6, then the rule says it has to depend on the left neighbor and right neighbor the resultant state is 1.0,1.0,0.6.

In the third state, it says depending on the left neighbor, so the resultant state is 1.0,1.0,1.0 is the attractor basin, which contains the class label.

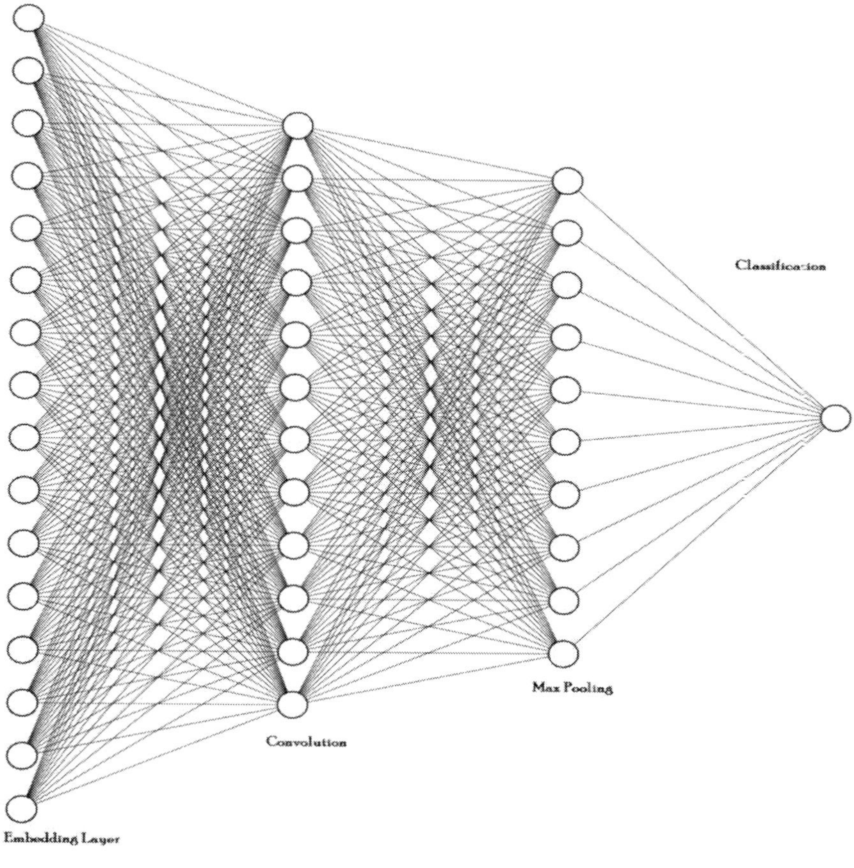

Figure 4. Design of CNN.

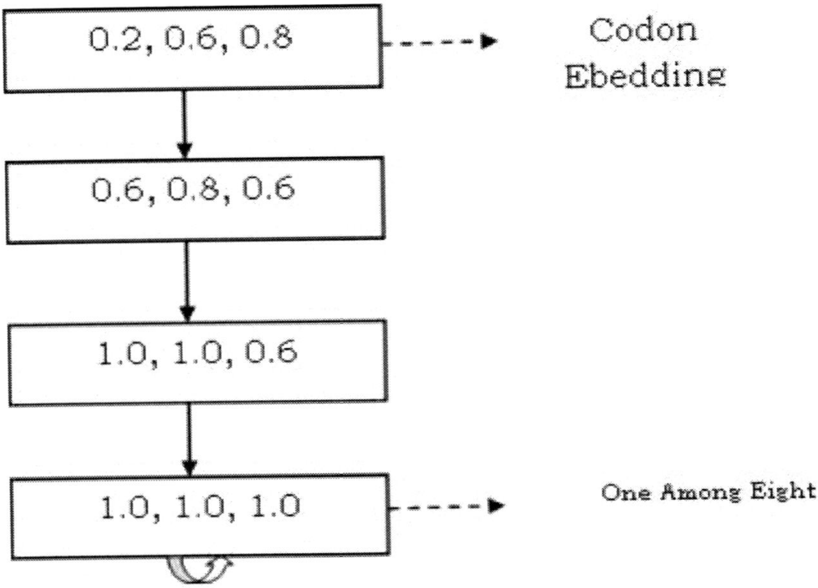

Figure 5. Working of NLCA.

Results and Discussion

Protein Coding Region Prediction (PCR)

PCR prediction is one of the most challenging problems addressed by many researchers. As we have earlier discussed, if we successfully predict whether the DNA sequence contains PCR or not, we can extract lots of information. This is the first method to apply PCR to predict these three chronic diseases. Many data sets are collected from totaling 10, 16,189, as reported in Table 3.

DLCDI initially takes a DNA sequence and predicts the PCR with boundaries, as shown below, with the strand types and type of exons also. We have identified c4.5, SPRINT, CART, N.N. as the potential models to predict PCR from the extensive literature survey done.

Table 3. Data Sets from US Center for Disease Control for PCR prediction

Data Set	Genomic 54	Genomic 108	Genomic 162	Genomic 252	Genomic 354
Training(Coding)	42,588	9,286	8,599	20,689	9,562
Training(Non Coding)	3,28,545	60,298	97,596	29,902	6,692
Testing(Coding)	54,856	9,794	7,588	9,895	3,901
Testing(Non Coding)	3,33,145	68,193	75,762	57,456	10,505

HUMAN sequence:

AAAAAGGGACCCCCAAAAAAAAAAGGGGGGGGGGGGG GGGGGAGGGCTTGGAAGTCTTGGGAGATTCACCTTTACTCAGA TGGTTGTTTACCTGTCTCGTGCACAGCTTGACACTTGGACTTTA AAGTGAGGATAAAGAACGACGAGGATGG

Exon Type	Left and Right Boundary		Strand Type
Internal	96	88	-
Internal	86	91	+
First	86	99	-
Internal	61	88	+
Internal	61	88	+
Terminal	61	117	+
Terminal	61	130	+
First	86	117	+
Terminal	86	130	+
Terminal	113	117	+
Internal	98	124	-
Internal	98	124	-
Internal	98	124	+
Internal	82	124	-
Terminal	94	124	+
Internal	78	124	-
Internal	94	124	-

We have compared the achieved model accuracy reported after processing the above datasets, as shown in Figure 6. The main strength of DLCDI is the CNN layer augmented with non-linear cellular automata rules. DLCDI reports a significantly lower error rate, i.e., 14.6%, compared with standard models cited in the literature. The model accuracy is also registered as 88.9%, which is considerably better compared to the cited research.

Table 4. Sensitivity and specificity values

	C4.5	SPRINT	CART	NN	DLCDI
Se	0.794	0.75	0.88	0.89	0.91
Sp	0.701	0.72	0.79	0.85	0.92
Percentage Accuracy	69.75	69.8	70.7	78	88.9

We have computed true positives, true negatives, false positives, and false negatives to measure the efficiency of the developed system are represented in Figure 7. The sensitivity and specificity values are calculated as illustrated in Table 4.

The main focus of the research is how this common platform can address many problems in bioinformatics. So we have identified CNN based NLCA technique to predict PCR with higher accuracy, which can process any length of DNA sequence and can process large data sets.

The second focus is adaptability; in order to test the flexibility of the system, we have downloaded DNA sequences from Fickett and Tung to test our method to predict PCR. The accuracy reported by our approach compared to the cited research is represented in Figure 8.

We have successfully achieved our primary goal of the research, i.e., to build a versatile, robust classifier to predict the protein-coding regions. In the next section, we will apply the developed classifier to predict the three chronic diseases.

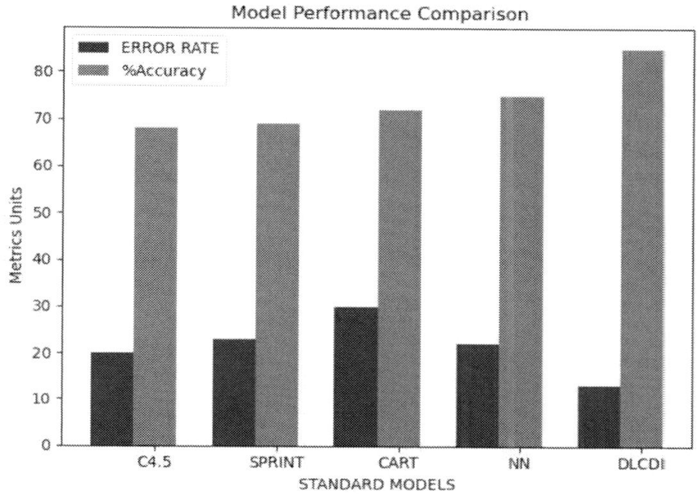

Figure 6. Model Accuracy Comparision of DLCDI.

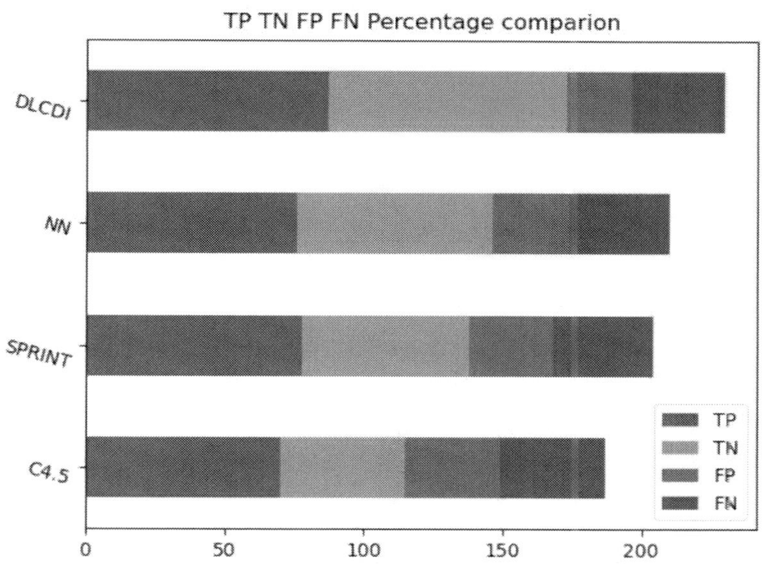

Figure 7. System Efficiency Comparision.

Cancer Prediction through DLCDI

Cancer prediction is one of the complex problems faced by many researchers. We have identified that if a DNA sequence contains PCR, then it can hold a promoter region. If the promoter region is placed, we can quickly assess whether the DNA sequence can likely have traces of cancer or not. After predicting the PCR promoter region is identified by NLCA, the process is explained below.

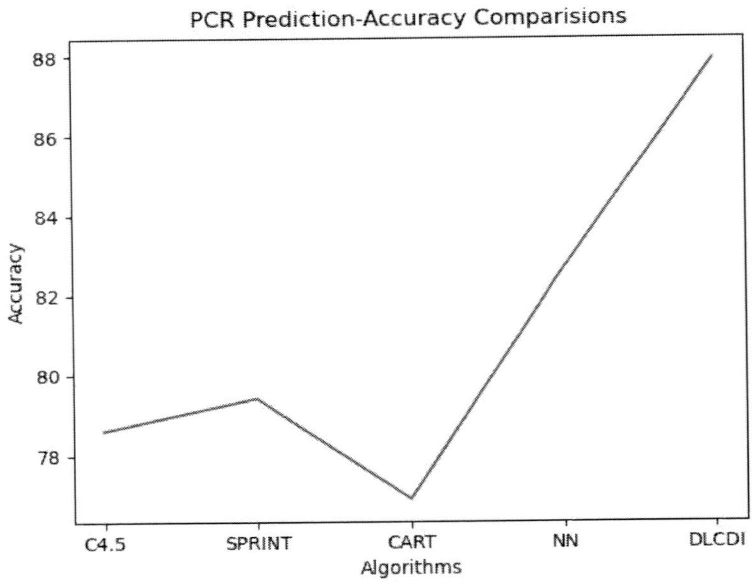

Figure 8. PCR prediction for Fickett and Tounge Datasets.

Sample Output of NLCA

>filtered DNA/PS sequence consisting of 449 residues.

MEKVNEERDAVFEDHIGDRRRSVRSLLEEAFADEMEKTSYDV EVADTPQPHIPIRFRHPPIAGPVHDVFGDAIHDIFQKMMKRGQAV DFCHWVSHLIATEIDEKFSEVAFRDVQYNPDIYVTDSTTEAKKLF

NDKIWPAIDKILQQNAETCPILSEKWSGIHVSGDQLKGQRHKQED
RFLAYPNGQYMDRGEDPISVLAVFDGHGGHECSQYAAGHLWET
WLEVRKSRDPSDSLEDQLRKSLELLDERMTVRSVKECWKGGSTA
VCCAIDMDQKLMALAWLGDSPGYVMSNIEFRQLTRGHSPSDERE
ARRVEEAGGQLFVIGGELRVNGVLNLTRALGDVPGRPMISNEPET
CQVPIESSDYLVLLACDGISDVFNERDLYQLVEAFANDYPVEDYA
ELSRFICTKAIEAGSADNVSVVIGFLRPPQDVWKLMKHESDDEDS
DVTDEE

Percentage of A's in sequence: 0.3684210526315789
Percentage of C's in sequence: 0.10526315789473684
Percentage of T's in sequence: 0.05263157894736842
Percentage of G's in sequence: 0.19736842105263158
A start codon (ATG) appears in the DNA sequence. 1
>results for 13914 residue sequence "fasta" starting "cttgaaagtg"
>base 1
c
>base 5
a
>base 10 to 20
ggataaaatcg
>base 13914
a

We have compared the developed classifier with the cited literature, i.e., big data analytics [21], predictive data mining [22], improved feature section method [23], and statistical computation method [24]. DLCDI has reported an accuracy of 81.23 with an error rate of less than 8%, which is far better compared with exiting standard methods, as shown in fig 9. The time is taken to compute whether the DNA sequence contains traces of cancer is 0.7 nanoseconds is far less compared to the existing literature. We have also calculated the overhead on the classifier to predict cancer traces, which is considerably less as the model efficiently uses the hybrid rules for classification.

Heart Disease/Attack Prediction through DLCDI

Once PCR was computed, a method called strand computation is proposed to predict the disease-causing symptoms in the heart.

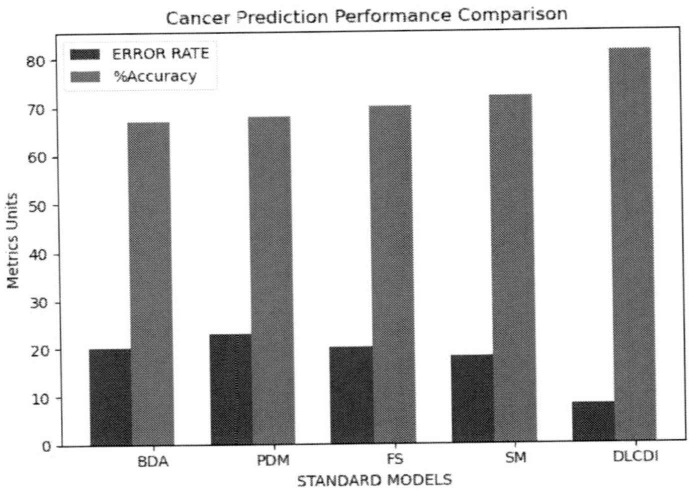

Figure 9. Cancer Prediction Accuracy Comparisons.

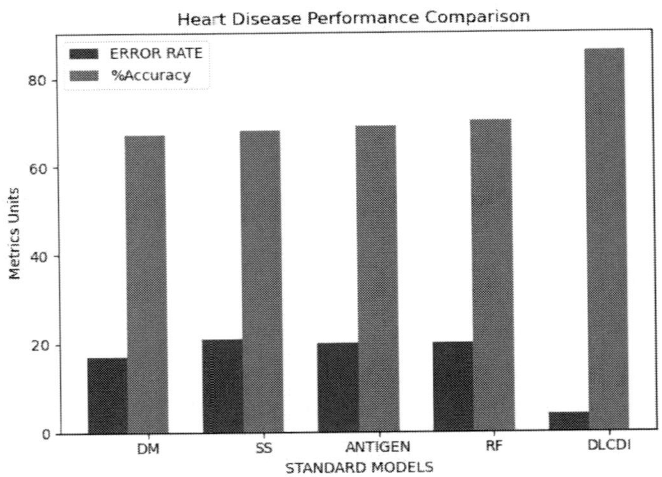

Figure 10. Heart Disease Prediction Accuracy Comparisons.

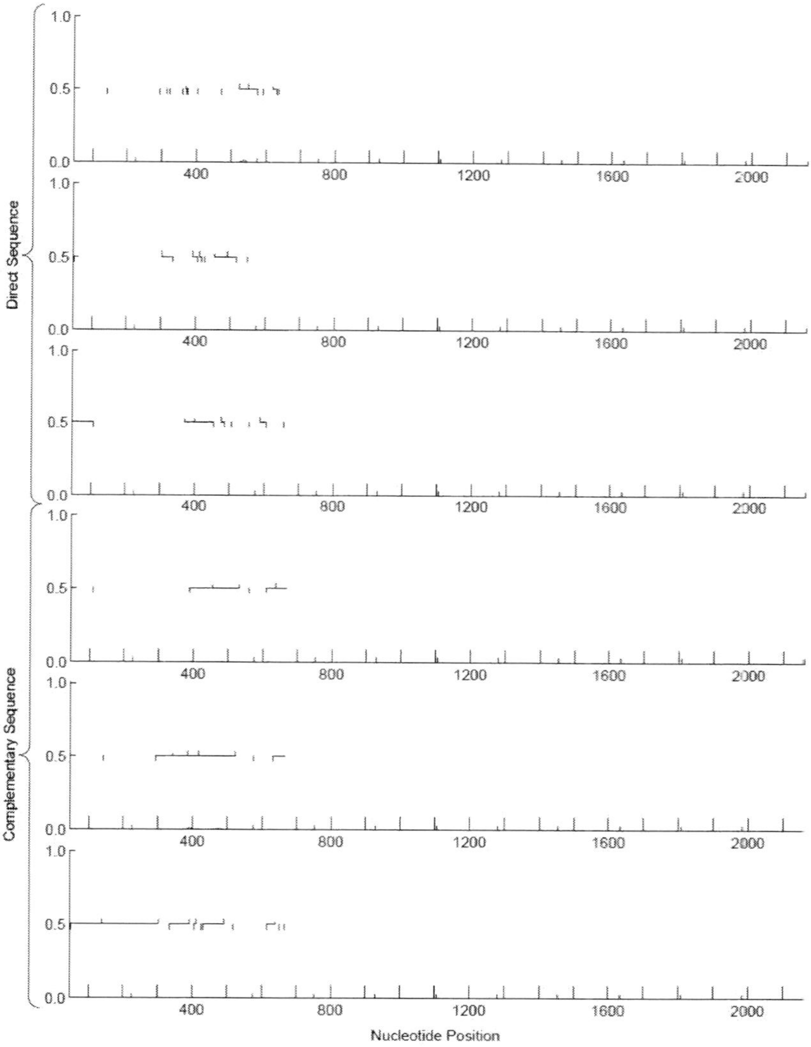

Figure 11. Strand Computation.

Strand computation class classifies the entire DNA strands into two, i.e., direct sequence and complementary sequence with six strands, as shown in Figure 11 with nucleotide positions to accurately analyze the disease growth rate. In nucleotide position, there is a chance of getting a heart attack.

The strand values are taken from 0 to1, which represent the probability values. Figure 11 shows all six strands between 0 to 600th. We have compared the developed classifier for heart disease prediction with the cited literature, i.e., Data Mining Method [25], Scoring System Method [26], Antigen Computation method [27], and risk computation method [28]. DLCDI has reported accuracy of 85.78 with an error rate of less than 4%, which is better compared with exiting standard methods, as shown in Figure 10.

Diabetes -II Prediction through DLCDI

Once PCR was computed, a process called mean analysis is proposed to predict whether the DNA sequence contains any symptoms of Diabetes II or not. In mean analysis (M.A.), the input is counted to identify the number of ATG/AAG/ATT in the sequences. As the neighbors keep on changing for the DNA sequence, M.A. has to predict the certainty of this sequence converting into an amino sequence. Based on the analysis of M.A., we can find whether the lines contain symptoms of diabetes or not.

Sample Output of MA

1 AAAAAAAAAA AAAAAATGAT GAAAAAAAAG GGGGGGGGGG GGGGGGGGGG GGGGGGGGGG

61 GCCCCCCCCC CCCCCCATGC CCCCCCCCCC CCCCATGCCC CCCCTTTTAA AAAAAAAAAA

121 AAAAAAAAAA AAAAAAAAAA AGGGGGGGGG GGGGGGGCAT G

ATG NO	Certainty factor	Frame No	Start Codon	End Codon	Amino Sequence
1	0.13	1	No	Yes	MMKKKGGGGGGGGG GAPPPPHAPPPPHAPPF KKKKKKKKKKKGGG GGA
3	0.10	2	No	No	MPPPPPMPPLLKKKKK KKKKKKGGGGGH
5	0.06	3	No	No	M
4	0.04	2	No		MPPLLKKKKKKKKKK KGGGGGH
2	0.04	1	No		MKKKGGGGGGGGGG APPPPHAPPPPHAPFFK KKKKKKKKKKGGGG GA

We have compared the developed classifier for diabetes prediction with the cited literature, i.e., Insulin Resistance Method [29], Offspring Study Method [30], and risk factor identification method [31]. DLCDI has reported accuracy of 89.76 with an error rate of less than 3%, better than exiting standard methods, as shown in Figure 12.

We have identified C4.5, SPRINT, CART, N.N. methods that can also be used to predict the chronic diseases individually, implemented them, and compared their results with our classifier DLCDI as shown in Figur 13. It is evident from the Figure that DLCDI is consistently reporting a better accuracy even with the cited specialized individual models. The time required to compute whether the developed classifier contains PCR or not for a DNA sequence of avg length 1024 is 0.66 nanoseconds. For cancer prediction, heart disease prediction, diabetes prediction, it consumes 0.7, 0.76, 0.79 nanoseconds, respectively, whereas, for PCR computation itself, it requires 0.8512 nanoseconds for the best methods cited in this chapter. As the classifier uses the best pooling, convolution techniques augmented with C.A. rules, the overhead of the classifier is significantly less. The efficiency of our method is measured by specificity and sensitivity, which is better compared to the existing literature.

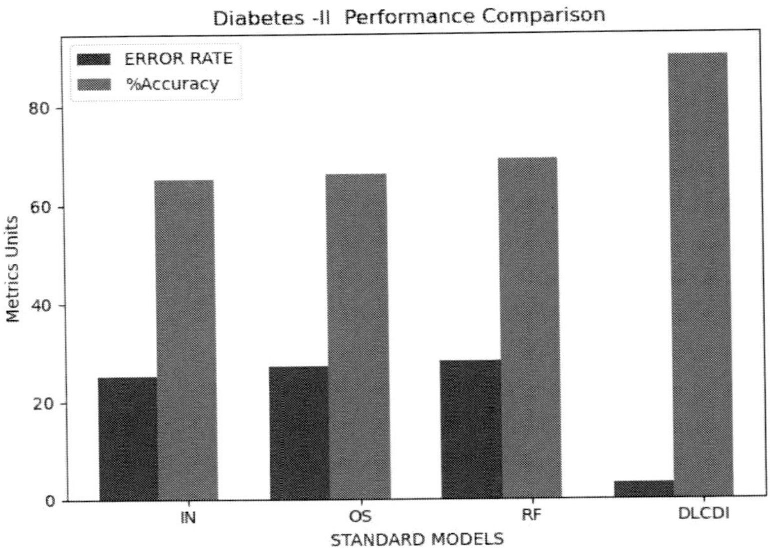

Figure 12. Diabetes II Prediction Accuracy Comparisons.

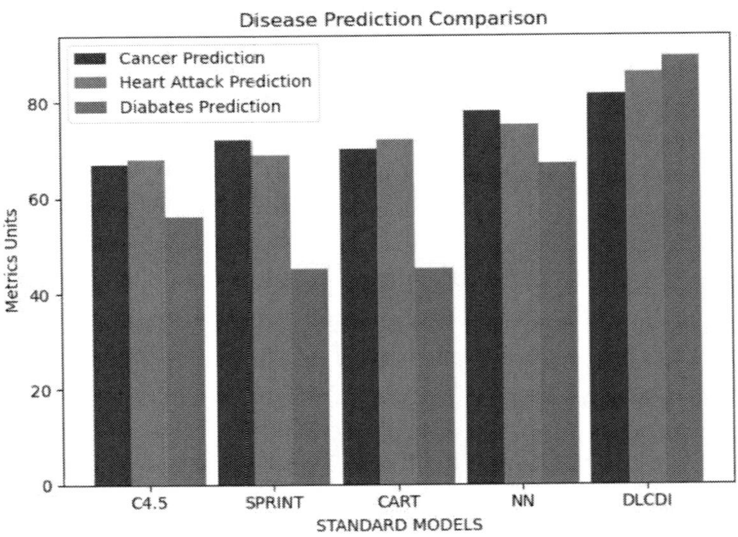

Figure 13. Chronic Disease Prediction using DLCDI.

We have identified C4.5, SPRINT, CART, N.N. methods that can also be used to predict the chronic diseases individually, implemented them, and compared their results with our classifier DLCDI as shown in Figure 13. It is evident from the Figure that DLCDI is consistently reporting a better accuracy even with the cited specialized individual models. The time required to compute whether the developed classifier contains PCR or not for a DNA sequence of avg length 1024 is 0.66 nanoseconds. For cancer prediction, heart disease prediction, diabetes prediction, it consumes 0.7, 0.76, 0.79 nanoseconds, respectively, whereas, for PCR computation itself, it requires 0.8512 nanoseconds for the best methods cited in this chapter. As the classifier uses the best pooling, convolution techniques augmented with C.A. rules, the overhead of the classifier is significantly less. The efficiency of our method is measured by specificity and sensitivity, which is better compared to the existing literature.

As we understood, PCR (Protein Coding Region) prediction is vital for identifying chronic diseases. We have compared DLCDI with the best available literature. C4.5 has the strength of adaptability, and the time it has processed to find the PCR is significantly less compared to SPRINT also. SPRINT has many advantages over C4.5, like divergence, the convergence of the input feasibility but lacks in the subsidized adaptability. Compared to C4.5, SPRINT, CART is a better option for the practitioners whose DNA sequences of lengths are less than 54bps. N.N. classifier stood as the best classifier to process datasets of large scales with an accuracy of 82.3%. N.N. is also adaptable as C4.5. We after implementing the existing literature, the specificity and sensitivity of DLCDI are better compared with all the other literature.

We have also considered the datasets for cancer prediction. We have taken a traditional BDA algorithm which gives an average accuracy of 65%, where the strength of it lies in processing more dynamic parameters. PDM algorithm was pronounced as the better algorithm compared to BDA as the specificity and sensitivity of this are better. F.S. reports a better accuracy handling with diverse parameters static and dynamics. S.M. algorithm was the best till the invention of DLCDI. Our algorithm says the accuracy of 78% for bipolar static and dynamic parameters.

CONCLUSION

We have successfully developed a mechanism to identify various chronic diseases. This mechanism was trained to predict the protein-coding regions first and then based on PCR to detect the disorders later. The classifier DLCDI was built on CNN augmented with cellular automata, which was robust and able to process large datasets of variable lengths. DLCDI was the first classifier from which chronic diseases are predicted. The classifier is thoroughly trained and tested with standard datasets and reports an average accuracy of 88.9%. This can be termed as the fastest classifier to predict PCR within 0.7 nanoseconds. The system's performance was measured with various parameters like time for computation, overhead, specificity, and sensitivity. DLCDI performance was compared with individual methods to predict cancer, heart attack, diabetes, and our classifier have reported an 8.2 to 12.6% increase in the average prediction accuracy. The above classifier can be extended to identify more chronic diseases like chronic lung disease, Alzheimer's, Kidney diseases, etc., by incorporating specific methods for fast computing.

REFERENCES

Alexander, Cheryl Ann, and Lidong Wang. 2017. *Big Data Analytics in Heart Attack Prediction.* https://doi.org/10.4172/2167-1168.1000393.

Al-Yasriy, Hamdalla F., Muayed S. Al-Husieny, Furat Y. Mohsen, Enam A. Khalil, and Zainab S. Hassan. 2020. "Diagnosis of Lung Cancer Based on C.T. Scans Using CNN." *In IOP Conference Series:*

Materials Science and Engineering. Vol. 928. IOP Publishing Ltd. https://doi.org/10.1088/1757-899X/928/2/022035.

Boulent, Justine, Samuel Foucher, Jérôme Théau, and Pierre Luc St-Charles. 2019. "Convolutional Neural Networks for the Automatic Identification of Plant Diseases." *Frontiers in Plant Science*. Frontiers Media S.A. https://doi.org/10.3389/fpls.2019.00941.

Chicco, Davide. 2017. *"Ten Quick Tips for Machine Learning in Computational Biology."* BioData Mining. BioMed Central Ltd. https://doi.org/10.1186/s13040-017-0155-3.

Cruz, Joseph A., and David S. Wishart. 2006. *"Applications of Machine Learning in Cancer Prediction and Prognosis."* Cancer Informatics. Libertas Academica Ltd. https://doi.org/10.1177/117693510600200030.

Danaee, Padideh, Reza Ghaeini, and David A. Hendrix. 2017. "A Deep Learning Approach for Cancer Detection and Relevant Gene Identification." *In Pacific Symposium on Biocomputing*, 0:219–29. World Scientific Publishing Co. Pte Ltd. https://doi.org/10.1142/9789813207813_0022.

Deng, Li, and Dong Yu. 2013. "Deep Learning: Methods and Applications." *Foundations and Trends in Signal Processing*. Now Publishers Inc. https://doi.org/10.1561/2000000039.

Gavhane, Aditi, Gouthami Kokkula, Isha Pandya, and Prof Kailas Devadkar. 2018. "Prediction of Heart Disease Using Machine Learning." In *Proceedings of the 2nd International Conference on Electronics, Communication and Aerospace Technology, ICECA* 2018, 1275–78. Institute of Electrical and Electronics Engineers Inc. https://doi.org/10.1109/ICECA.2018.8474922.

Holzinger, Andreas. 2016. "Interactive Machine Learning for Health Informatics: When Do We Need the Human-in-the-Loop?" *Brain Informatics* 3 (2): 119–31. https://doi.org/10.1007/s40708-016-0042-6.

Iqbal, Muhammad Javed, Zeeshan Javed, Haleema Sadia, Ijaz A. Qureshi, Asma Irshad, Rais Ahmed, Kausar Malik, et al. 2021. "Clinical Applications of Artificial Intelligence and Machine

Learning in Cancer Diagnosis: Looking into the Future." *Cancer Cell International.* BioMed Central Ltd. https://doi.org/10.1186/s12935-021-01981-1.

Krithiga, R., and P. Geetha. 2020. "Deep Learning Based Breast Cancer Detection and Classification Using Fuzzy Merging Techniques." *Machine Vision and Applications* 31 (7–8). https://doi.org/10.1007/s00138-020-01122-0.

Lai, Hang, Huaxiong Huang, Karim Keshavjee, Aziz Guergachi, and Xin Gao. 2019. "Predictive Models for Diabetes Mellitus Using Machine Learning Techniques." *BMC Endocrine Disorders* 19 (1). https://doi.org/10.1186/s12902-019-0436-6.

Martin-Isla, Carlos, Victor M. Campello, Cristian Izquierdo, Zahra Raisi-Estabragh, Bettina Baeßler, Steffen E. Petersen, and Karim Lekadir. 2020. "Image-Based Cardiac Diagnosis With Machine Learning: A Review." *Frontiers in Cardiovascular Medicine. Frontiers Media S.A.* https://doi.org/10.3389/fcvm.2020.00001.

Mostavi, Milad, Yu Chiao Chiu, Yufei Huang, and Yidong Chen. 2020. "Convolutional Neural Network Models for Cancer Type Prediction Based on Gene Expression." *BMC Medical Genomics 13* (April). https://doi.org/10.1186/s12920-020-0677-2.

Naz, Huma, and Sachin Ahuja. 2020. "Deep Learning Approach for Diabetes Prediction Using PIMA Indian Dataset." *Journal of Diabetes and Metabolic Disorders* 19 (1): 391–403. https://doi.org/10.1007/s40 200-020-00520-5.

Ravi, Daniele, Charence Wong, Fani Deligianni, Melissa Berthelot, Javier Andreu-Perez, Benny Lo, and Guang Zhong Yang. 2017. "Deep Learning for Health Informatics." *IEEE Journal of Biomedical and Health Informatics* 21 (1): 4–21. https://doi.org/10.1109/JBHI.20 16.2636665.

Sajja, Tulasi Krishna, and Hemantha Kumar Kalluri. 2020. "A Deep Learning Method for Prediction of Cardiovascular Disease Using Convolutional Neural Network." *Revue d'Intelligence Artificielle 34* (5): 601–6. https://doi.org/10.18280/ria.340510.

Shah, Devansh, Samir Patel, and Santosh Kumar Bharti. 2020. "Heart Disease Prediction Using Machine Learning Techniques." *S.N. Computer Science* 1 (6): 345. https://doi.org/10.1007/s42979-020-00365-y.

Shankar, VirenViraj, Varun Kumar, Umesh Devagade, Vinay Karanth, and K. Rohitaksha. 2020. "Heart Disease Prediction Using CNN Algorithm." *S.N. Computer Science* 1 (3). https://doi.org/10.1007/s42979-020-0097-6.

Shouman, Mai, Tim Turner, and Rob Stocker. 2011. *"Using Decision Tree for Diagnosing Heart Disease Patients."* https://doi.org/10.5555/ 24836 28.2483633.

Sneha, N., and Tarun Gangil. 2019. "Analysis of Diabetes Mellitus for Early Prediction Using Optimal Features Selection." *Journal of Big Data 6 (1).* https://doi.org/10.1186/s40537-019-0175-6.

Soguero-Ruiz, Cristina, Inmaculada Mora-Jiménez, Miguel A. Mohedano-Munoz, Manuel Rubio-Sanchez, Pablo De Miguel-Bohoyo, and Alberto Sanchez. 2020. "Visually Guided Classification Trees for Analyzing Chronic Patients." *BMC Bioinformatics 21* (March). https://doi.org/10.1186/s12859-020-3359-3.

Sree, Pokkuluri Kiran, and S. S.S.N.Usha Devi Nedunuri. 2020. "A Novel Cellular Automata Classifier for COVID-19 Trend Prediction." *Journal of Health Sciences 10* (1): 34–38. https://doi.org/10.17532/ jhsci.2020.907.

Xiao, Xuan, Guang Fu Xue, Biljana Stamatovic, and Wang Ren Qiu. 2020. "Using Cellular Automata to Simulate Domain Evolution in Proteins." *Frontiers in Genetics 11.* https://doi.org/10.3389/fgene.2020.00515.

Xie, Juanying, Ran Liu, Joseph Luttrell, and Chaoyang Zhang. 2019. "Deep Learning Based Analysis of Histopathological Images of Breast Cancer." *Frontiers in Genetics* 10 (FEB). https://doi.org/10.3389/ fgene.2019.00080.

Yadav, Dhyan Chandra, and Saurabh Pal. 2020. "Prediction of Thyroid Disease Using Decision Tree Ensemble Method." *Human-Intelligent*

Systems Integration 2 (1–4): 89–95. https://doi.org/10.1007/s42454-020-00006-y.

Yadav, Samir S., Shivajirao M. Jadhav, Snigdha Nagrale, and Niraj Patil. 2020. "Application of Machine Learning for the Detection of Heart Disease." In 2nd International Conference on Innovative Mechanisms for Industry Applications, ICIMIA 2020 - Conference Proceedings, 165–72. *Institute of Electrical and Electronics Engineers Inc.* https://doi.org/10.1109/ICIMIA48430.2020.9074954.

Zhou, Huaping, Raushan Myrzashova, and Rui Zheng. 2020. "Diabetes Prediction Model Based on an Enhanced Deep Neural Network." *Eurasip Journal on Wireless Communications and Networking 2020* (1). https://doi.org/10.1186/s13638-020-01765-7.

In: Intelligent Information Retrieval … ISBN: 978-1-68507-301-5
Editors: Parma Nand et al. © 2021 Nova Science Publishers, Inc.

Chapter 5

NOVEL APPROACH TO HEALTH MONITORING SYSTEM

Amrit Muskan*, Kanishka, Karan Malhotra, Nishi Kumari, Manisha Rajoriya and Usha Tiwari
Department of Electrical Electronics and Communication Engineering
School of Engineering and Technology, Sharda University,
Greater Noida UP, India

ABSTRACT

An essential part of our life is Internet, and it has allowed machines or devices that we use in our daily life to be monitored via IoT technology. A sector that has seen an immense amount of growth because of IoT is the health sector. For example, suppose that if someone is suffering from some heart disease, his/her Heart Rate, Body Temperature, etc., can be easily measured on the application. The customized Android application can measure all these things of the patient that should be under observation. The sensors in these devices constantly measure all the changes and immediately alert the doctor as well as to the family members as a Notification. In this way, the patient can live in their own environment and live their lives freely and peacefully. This chapter reviews various approaches that have been

* Corresponding Author's E-mail: muskanamrit56@gmail.com.

done in this field. It discusses designs and methodologies carried out in the past concerning the use of android applications in Heart health.

Keywords: Internet of Things (IoT), blynk application, smart health, pulse sensor, temperature sensor

INTRODUCTION

- The Internet of Things (IoT) is introduced by Kevin Aston in 1999 [1]. IoT is a communication medium in which it is connected to each other or maybe other more extensive networks.
- The network collects all the necessary information and uses it for our benefit. Currently, almost 20 Billion devices are using IoT, and it is assumed that there will be 75 billion devices by 2025 [3].
- The Next Generation Cities would be Smart and would use IoT. Life would be very easy in these cities. The Department of Health is improving day by day, but because of the lack of resources, people living in rural areas cannot access these facilities [8].

People in rural areas can't afford these devices as they are expensive. These devices can track all of human activities, keep track of it, and work on the progress of human beings. It is beneficial for us as we can live in our own surroundings and can still be monitored by the doctors.

- If something wrong happens, it will immediately ping the Doctor and the Family with a notification. IoT is generally something that will change our lives forever [10, 11].
- Thanks to IoT, the information can be shared anywhere across the world, increasing the speed of recovery and providing medical facilities. The downside to it is real-time analyses, and the estimates are not proper [13, 14, 16].

All Thanks to the "Blynk application developer" created especially for "Smart Health," that shows real-time to time data and sends all the data to the doctor and the family of the patient. The principal reason for this is to provide patients the required medical help as soon as possible.

LITERATURE REVIEW

In order to come up with a presentable and well-defined smart monitoring system, a number of research papers have been reviewed and summarized in this section.

According to the World Health Organisation, Health is a global issue for humanity. In the last decade, health, according to the World Health Organization, is a worldwide concern that affects all of humankind. The topic of Health Monitoring System has experienced a considerable rise in the study over the previous decade. The primary goal is to keep track of the patient's health. The technology would create a trustworthy and long-term patient monitoring software so that healthcare professionals may care for their patients virtually as well in real-time [10]. It is a mobile phone-based wireless health care monitoring system that gives real-time patient information and updates it in the cloud. The paper [11] discusses the cost, ease of use, accuracy, and data security of real-time heart monitoring systems.

The method facilitates contact between the doctor and the patients, allowing for stress-free communication [14] also shows a powerful IoT-based combination remote monitoring system. It keeps track of the patient's heart rate, breathing rate, and other vital health indicators.

We can now distribute health solutions with wisdom and estimate the power of existence used by individuals and medical institutions thanks to the current state of IoT. The use of network edge gate methods to deliver high-quality services such as embedded, localized data entry storage, and local data processing for smart eHealth is discussed in [6].

Smart cities, transportation, and health monitoring benefit from effective Internet of Things (IoT) use and power management. In [5] section, a description of power management, difficulties, and opportunities is provided, as well as a framework for energy efficiency and smart city planning based on IoT [4]. contains extensive technological study, agreements, and the construction of urban IoT.

The authors of [17] recruit current evolution in the field of wearable sensors and associated systems in the medical arena. Wireless monitoring utilizing wearable biomedical devices is expanding considerably these days. Remote monitoring systems can take advantage of wearable technologies. Similarly, [14] looked at ECG monitoring as a case study and focused on regenerating electronic real-time medical records in the future. According to [18], the majority of existing portable ECG devices need a smartphone application to function [10]. As a result, the authors propose a new ECG monitoring system that makes use of the Internet of Things. Wearables are used to capture ECG data, which is then tracked and sent to the cloud. The authors published a survey in [13] that compared low-cost and inefficient health monitoring technologies that have been described in recent years. The next generation is also introduced in the future.

We can conclude from the above literature that wearable devices, remote monitoring systems, and the internet of things are the future of the health sector and telemedicine. As a result, we present a novel approach to a smart health monitoring system capable of measuring a patient and any individual under surveillance.

METHODOLOGY

Parameters like Heart Rate Variability (HRV), Body Temperature (BT), and Heart Rate (HR), which are important indicators for heath check-up status, have immense diagnostic value. Up to this point, persistent observing of those physiological boundaries has been conceivable just inside the emergency clinic climate, and these days with the advancement of wearable innovation, these boundaries are frequently checked precisely, ceaselessly, and progressively [17].

Concept of PPG (Photoplethysmography)

Every human being has a different HR value. The number of heartbeats per minute and Beats Per Minute (BPM) is its unit. There are a lot of factors that affect the value of HR; they are listed as Body movements, Hunger, Toughness, Emotional state, Air temperature.

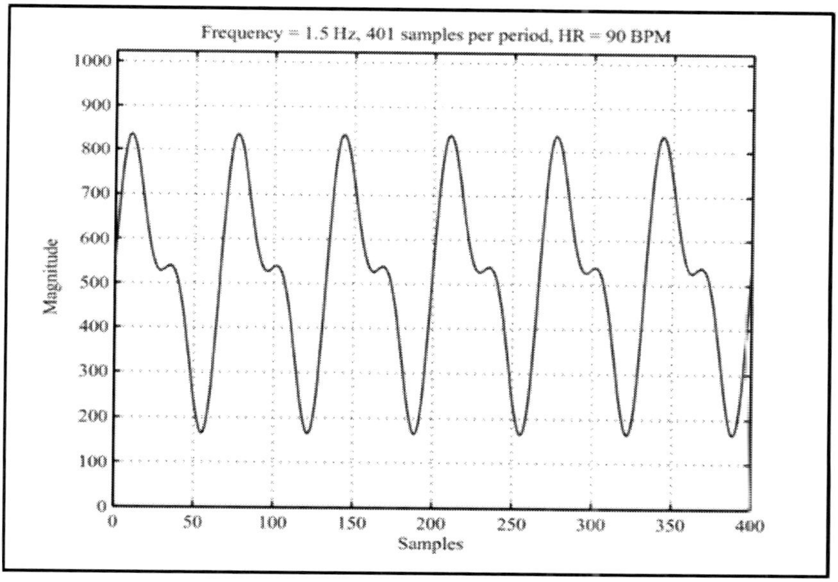

Figure 1. PPG signal.

For normal Humans, the value of HR is between 60 and 100. This might vary for athletes and sportspersons. PPG is the neural transmission architecture and the recording of electrical activity in the heart muscle.

Pulse Sensor

It has two sides; on one side, there is LED, and on the other side, we have some circuitry. The circuitry does the amplification and the noise cancellation. The LED is placed over a vein as there is blood flowing in the vein. We can easily monitor the flow of blood and heartbeats as well.

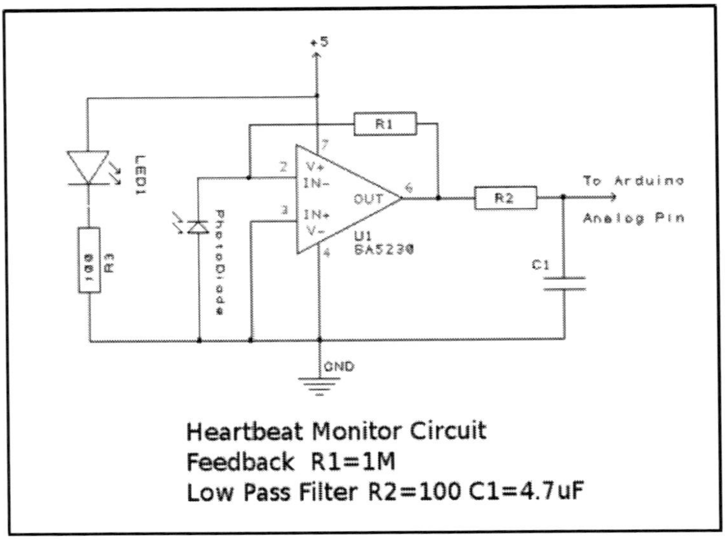

Figure 2. Pulse Sensor Circuit Diagram.

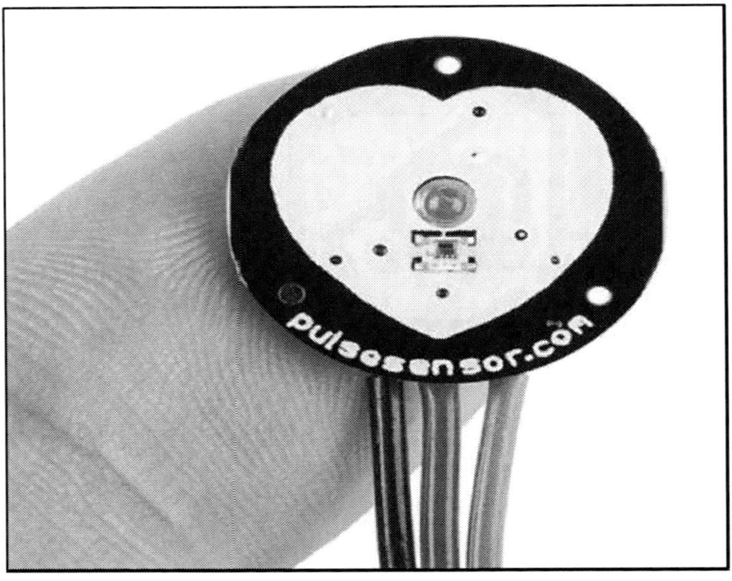

Figure 3. Pulse Sensor.

Applications of a Pulse Sensor

a) Sleep tracking
b) Anxiety monitoring
c) Remote patient monitor
d) Health bands
e) Advanced gaming consoles

Temperature Sensor

The DS18B20 Temperature Sensor conveys over a one-wire transport. It is a temperature sensor with a 12-bit ADC. It may be handily associated with an Arduino computerized input. The sensors have an accuracy in the range of -10 °C to the + 85 °C.

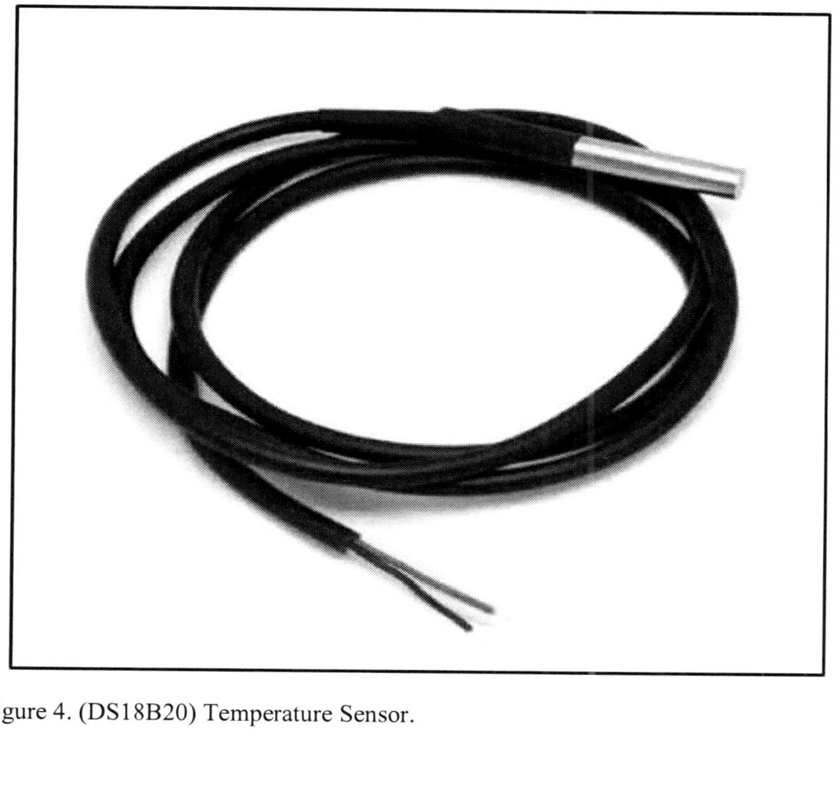

Figure 4. (DS18B20) Temperature Sensor.

Arduino Pro Mini Controller

It is an 8-bit microcontroller. It has a small size and because of that, it is used in battery-operated and portable operations. It has 14-optical I/O pins and can also use 6-pins as a Pulse Width Modulation (PWM) output and 6-pins for analog input.

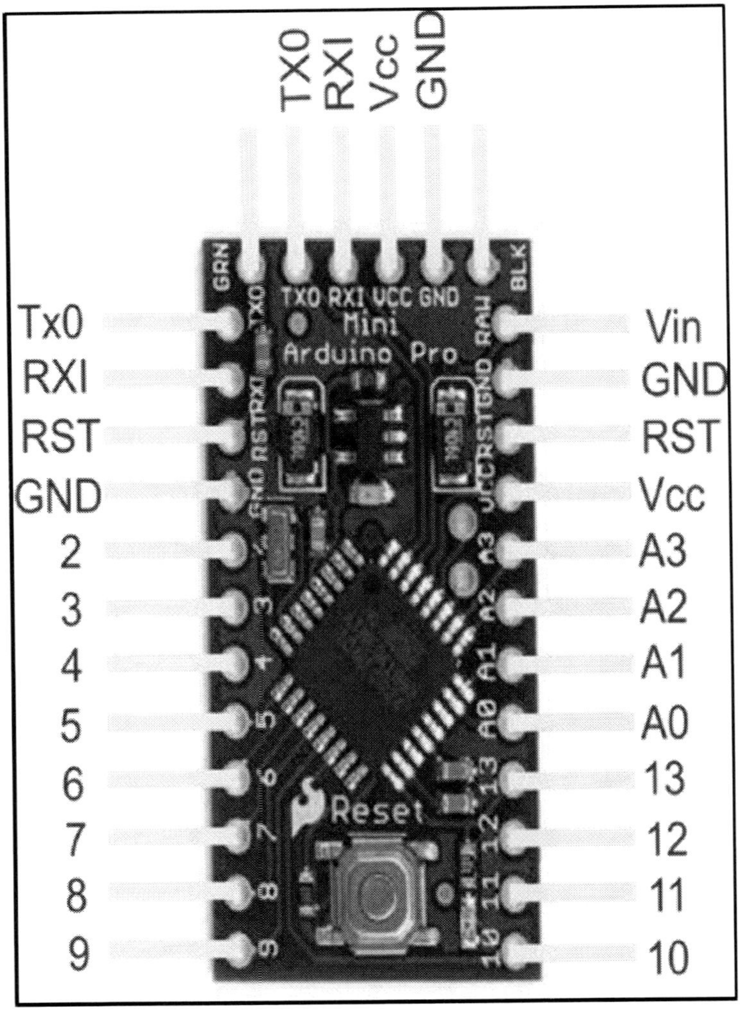

Figure 5. Arduino Pro Mini.

Table 1. Specifications of Arduino Pro Mini

About	Value
Program Memory	32kb
ADC Pin	16x10 Bit
IO current	40 mA
MCU	8-bit ATmega328p
Input/Output	14xDIO
Frequency	16MHz
Operating Voltage	5V

HC-06 Bluetooth Module

Bluetooth is a mode of communication that uses the 2.4-2.48 GHz frequency range. These are primarily for short-distance contact. The range for short-distance communication is usually 10 to 20m, not more than that. The distance can be increased to 100m by new technology mediums.

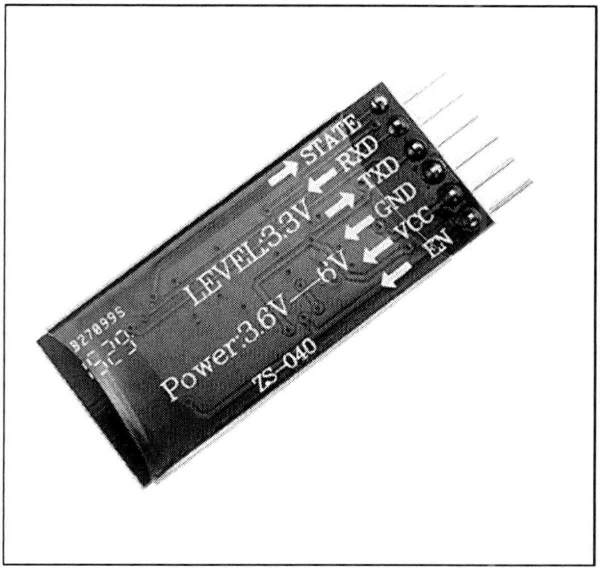

Figure 6. HC-06 Bluetooth Module.

The HC-06 Bluetooth module can only answer incoming link requests, and it cannot request connections from other Bluetooth modules.

Table 2. Specifications of HC-06 bluetooth module

About	Value
Synchronous Speed	1MBps/1MBps
Frequency	16 MHz
Communication frequency	2.4 GHz
Precision	≤ -80 dBm
Power Output	-4 / +6 dBm
Asynchronous Speed	2.1MBps/160 Kbps
Bluetooth Protocol	Bluetooth 2.0+EDR
Operating voltage	18.5v (3.3v)

ESP8266 Node MCU

This is a microcontroller that provides Wi-Fi capability. It requires an outer non-volatile capacity and a couple of antennas. There are various modules and advancement sheets. Some advancement sheets utilize fundamental ESP8266 modules, non-volatile storage, and in this way, the radio wire on the PCB.

The Node MCU is an improvement board associated with ESP8266 and firmware with a similar name. The Figure is of the Node MCU advancement board with an ESP8266 module patched to the PCB of the Node MCU. The advancement board requires circuits around the module; boot setup empower enable pin, pull-up and pull-down, the USB chip to associate the ESP8266 to the USB, and an auto reset circuit to empower the transfer device to put ESP8266 into the flashing mode. The 3.3 V power is changed over from the 5 V of USB for ESP8266.

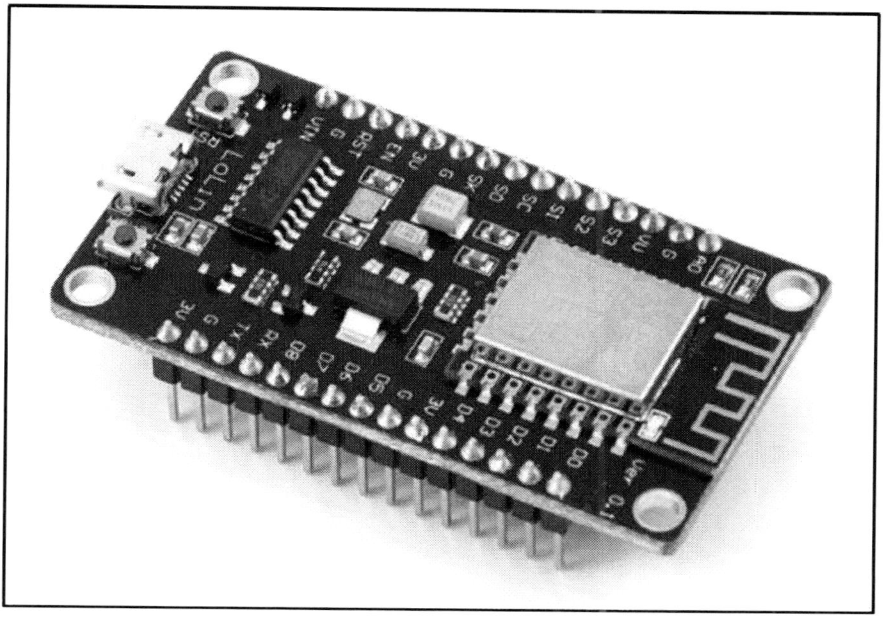

Figure 7. Node MCU.

Blynk Application for IOS/Android Users

This application is an IoT platform developed for android/IOS users. These are made so that controllers like Arduino can be controlled over the internet.

With the help of this app's graphical interface, it will take much less time to develop by using Widgets without having to write the actual code.

List of Widgets

a) Timer
b) Joystick
c) Gauge
d) Email

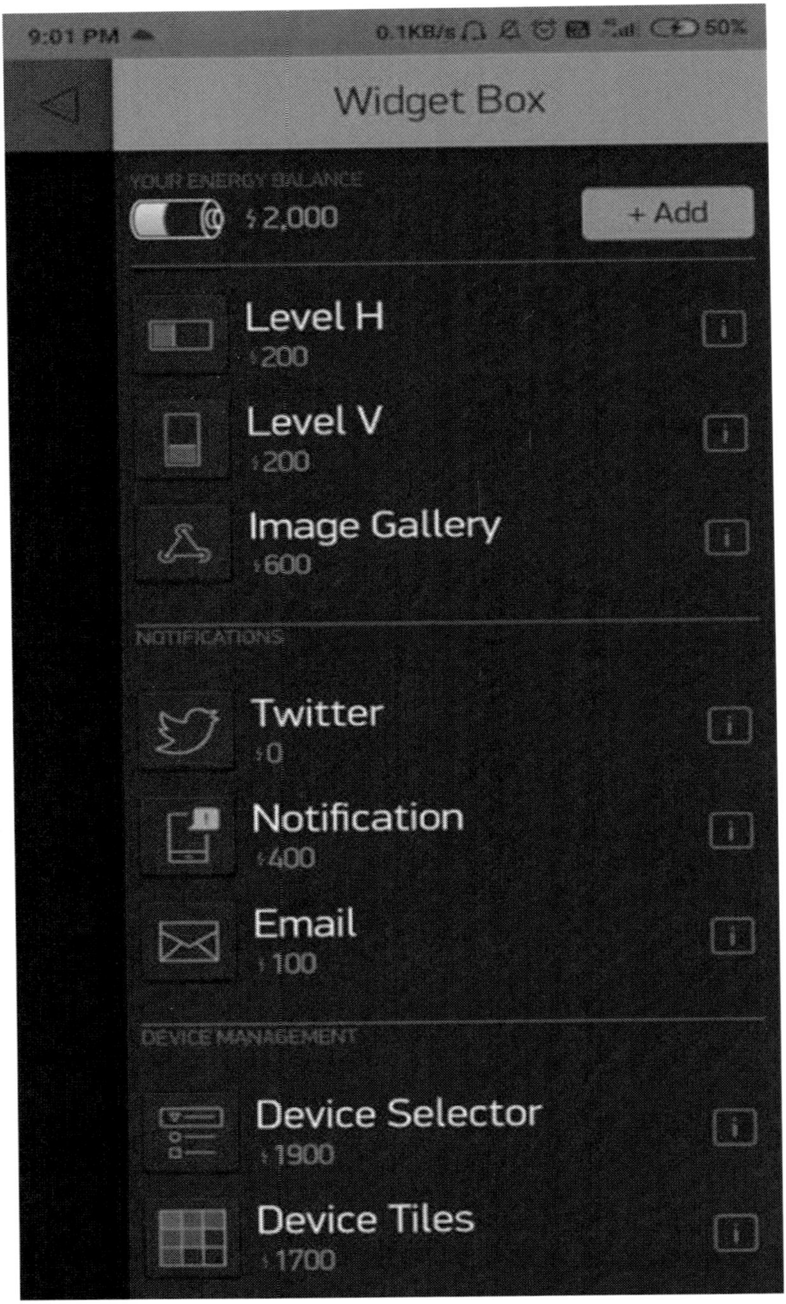

Figure 8. Blynk Application Widget Boxes.

Arduino Software

It is open-source that helps us in writing the codes; it makes it easier to upload it on board. It is available on platforms like Apple (MacOS X), Windows and etc.

The Java language is used to create the IDE and is called Processing or Wiring according to the language. You can easily access it from the internet by simply searching "Arduino Software IDE." The codes are written in C, C++ and java.

Advanced controllers which are compatible with Arduino Software are Blynk, ESP, Raspberry Pi, STM32. By consuming low energy online, Bluetooth functions can be used for closed circuit communications with the aid of the requirements of these controllers.

System Design/Architecture

It comprises of two sections:

- Hardware Design: - Components such as the Temperature Sensor, Pulse Sensor, Arduino UNO, and Wi-Fi shield ESP8266 are included.
- Software Design
  1) Arduino UNO: - It's an open-source architecture based on the ATmega 328P in essence. Arduino has 14-advanced Input/Output pins. It is a simple USB interface and 32kb flash memory used to store the codes like C. An ICSP header for directly interfacing the Arduino board as a sequential device and a reset button to reset the programs stored on the chip. PWM outputs can also be used with these 6-pins. An ADC is a system that transforms Analog data into Digital data. These pins on the Arduino board have an 'A' in front of the mark (A0 through A5) and can read the Analog voltages. The ADC on Arduino is a 10-bit converter that can precisely

perceive Analog values of 1024. This signifies that the voltage is anywhere between 0 and 5 volts; input voltages would be scheduled into integer values between the range values of 0 and 1023.

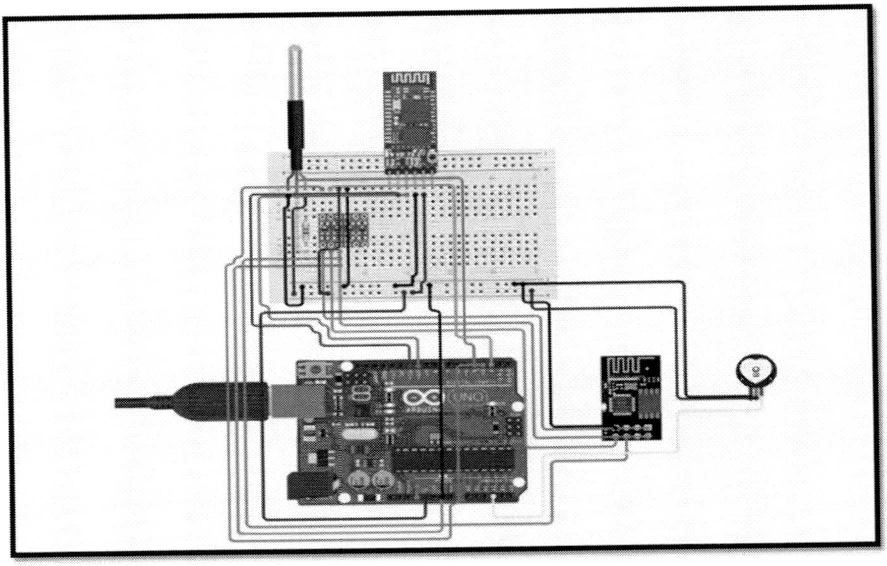

Figure 9. Circuit Diagram of Health Monitoring System.

2) NODE MCU: - It's an open-source IoT platform. This includes equipment based on ESP-12 and firmware running on the ESP8266 Wi-Fi SoC. The term "Node MCU" refers to the firmware; rather, they have development kits. The firmware uses the Lua scripting language. It uses several projects that are open source
3) KG011(Heartbeat Sensor): - The heartbeat sensor is based on the photo plethysmography (PPG) theory. As the volume of blood in each organ of the body increases, the light force in the vascular organ changes. The rate of heartbeat selects the rate of blood volume distribution because the blood absorbs light and the heartbeats are equal to the signal pulses.

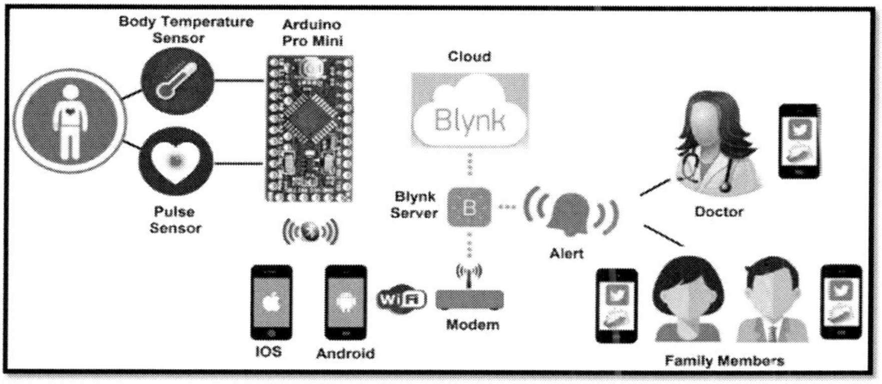

Figure 10. Proposed Structure of the System.

The pacing linked to the heartbeats is essential when the heartbeat rate is to be tracked.

Working of a Heartbeat Sensor

In order to recognize the finger's pulse, the heartbeat sensor is made up of Infrared LED and a photodiode. On the other hand, The Infrared LED is accessible on one side, and the photodiode is present on the other side. At the moment where the light source illuminates the tissue, the photodiode captures the reflecting rays. The detector output is an electrical signal that indicates how many pulses the sensor has counted. This pulse rate sensor has the following characteristics; LED for the heartbeat, Digital output, Compact with + 5 V DC operating voltage scale.

Result and Discussion

The result is presented on "Health Monitoring." Firstly, we install all the components on the breadboard for measuring Interbeat Interval (IBI) using PPG wave. After passing 50% of the wave signal through the microcontroller, IBI is measured. BPM is the average value of 10 IBM. For measuring the time between the heartbeats accurately high-resolution sampling is very important. For timer interrupt, 2ms frequency of 500Hz is obtained.

Analog value of the pulse sensor is obtained after this procedure. For correct amplitude measurement, the highest and the lowest value of the PPG must be determined. The thresh value is 512. Before the signal is updated to avoid false reading and noise the IBI value must be passed 3/5 times. If the threshold value is greater than 50% of the amplitude signal and its time duration is greater than 3/5 times the IBI, the values should be stored in the sequence of 10 elements.

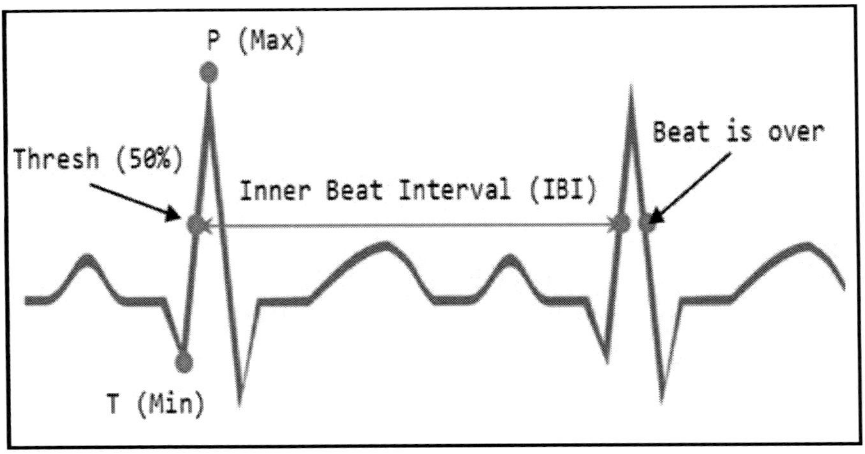

Figure 11a. Signal (PPG) for 2 consecutive hearts 11(b): -Signal (PPG) for consecutive hearts.

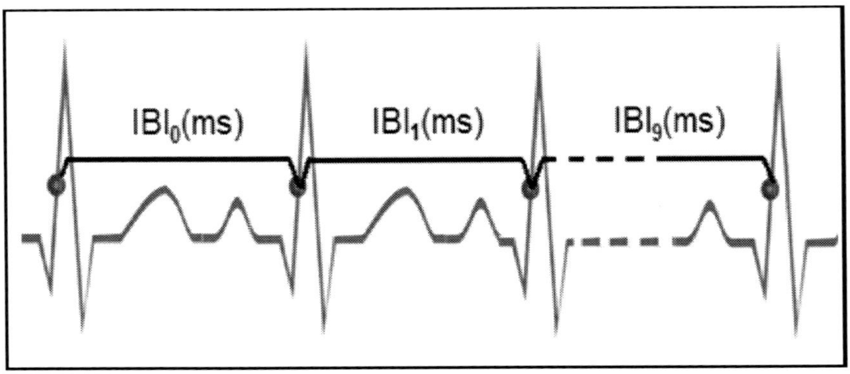

Figure 11b. Signal (PPG) for consecutive hearts.

$$IBI\ average = \frac{(IBI0 + IBI1 + \cdots IBI9)}{10} \tag{1}$$

$$BPM = \frac{60000}{IBI\ average} \tag{2}$$

The value of the BPM is determined in a millisecond by taking the average of the total IBI values, as shown in the figure 11(a), after a total of 10 successive IBI registrations. With the help of formula (i) and formula(ii) we can calculate IBI and BPM values. Hence, we install the BLYNK Application on the phones for sending the data by using ESP8266 (Node MCU).

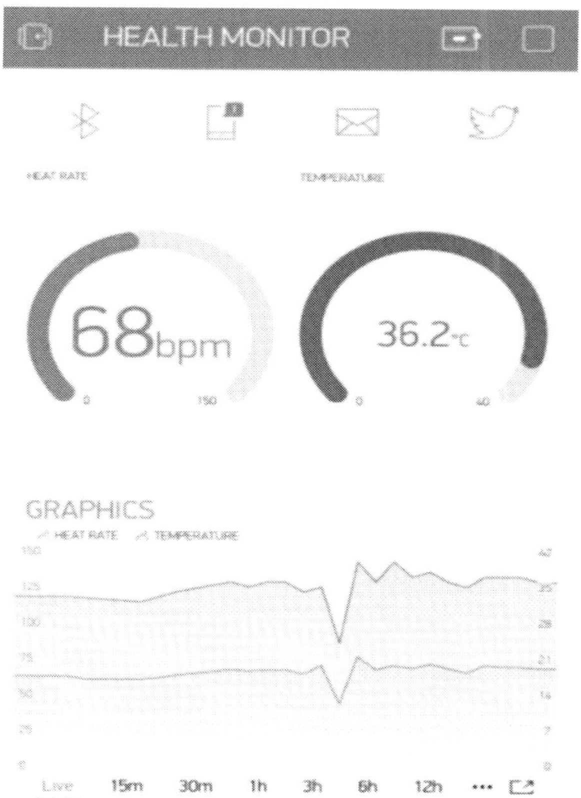

Figure 12a. There is an interface of the application.

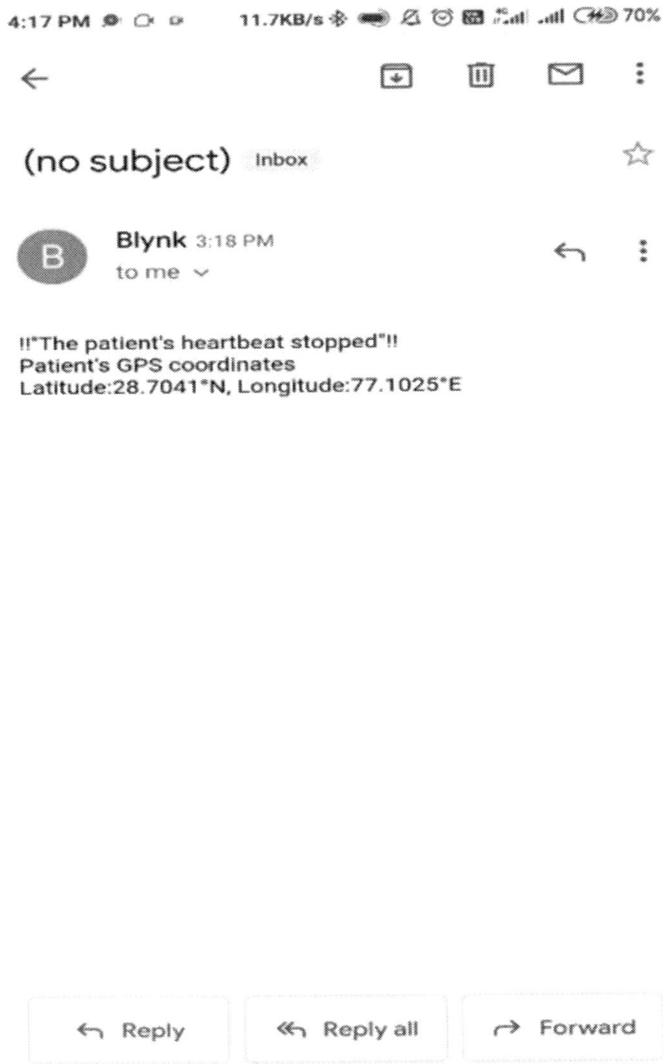

Figure 12b. The email has been sent to the doctors as well as to the family members.

In some significant cases, the application will send a notification of the patient's family members and the doctor.

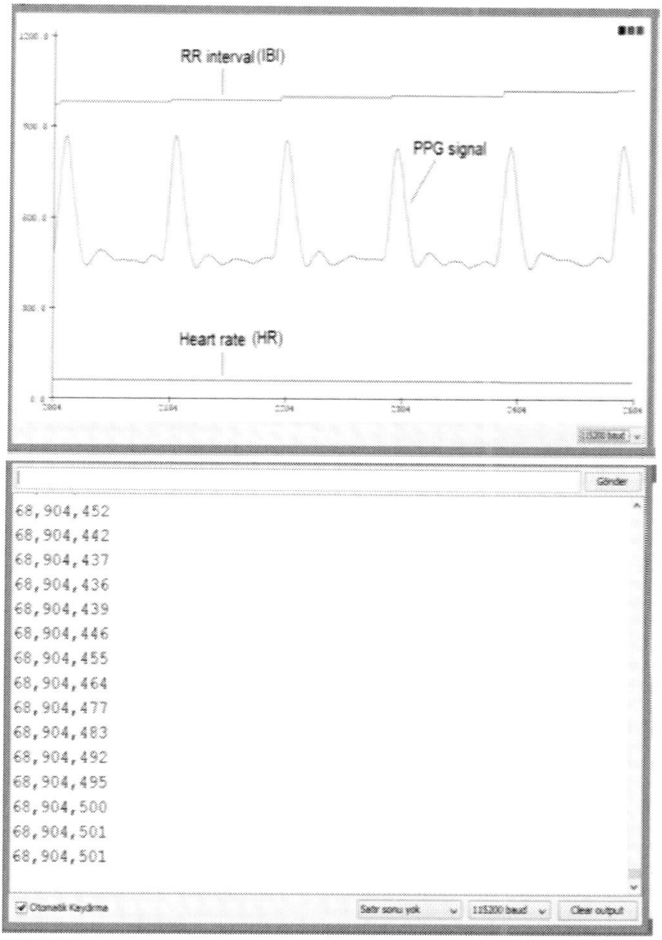

Figure 13. A real-time PPG signal is obtained from the Arduino IDE monitor and we can see the numeric values of HR, IBI and PPG signals.

CONCLUSION

Nowadays, IoT application is widely used in every sector. One of them is the fitness region and this region gives superb possibilities for us with new programs. The tracking of the sufferers, who have to be saved beneath regular surveillance, within the medical institution surroundings may be very hard with the current methods and infrastructures. The number of beds in the hospital is very less, so the patient suffers in many cases. Many fitness troubles that are supposed to be monitored fast may also cause critical troubles for the affected person since they cannot be monitored on time.

Early analysis is very crucial for patients with heart diseases. The advanced device constantly measures the coronary heart and temperatures of the patient and offers tracking and monitoring through an android based interface. When the affected person's critical facts reach a determined restriction value, the cell software indicates the affected person and the humans inside the region. This caution is made at a quantity degree that humans close to the affected person can hear.

If there may be no one inside the region of the affected person who can assist him, the affected person's coronary heartbeat, temperature, and coordination records are dispatched to their own family and doctor through Twitter and email notifications.

The fundamental cause of the instrument is to make an offer to get resources as soon as possible. So, there could be an all-encompassing possibility that the patient's stamina would not harm in the event of a potential heart attack soreness.

REFERENCES

[1] Ashton, K. That 'internet of things' thing *RFID journal*, 2009, 22(7), pp. 97-114.

[2] Gubbi, J., Buyya, R., Marusic, S., Palaniswami, M, Future generation computer systems, *Internet of Things (IoT): A vision, architectural elements, and future directions*, 2013, 29(7), pp. 1645-1660.

[3] Evans, D., CISCO white paper. *The internet of things: How the next evolution of the internet is changing everything,* 2011, 1, pp. 1-11.

[4] Zanella, A., Bui, N., Castellani, A., Vangelista, L., Zorzi, M. Internet of things for smart cities, *IEEE Internet of Things journal*, 2014, 1(1), pp. 22-32.

[5] Ejaz, W., Naeem, M., Shahid, A., Anpalagan, A., Jo, M Efficient energy management for the internet of things in smart cities, *IEEE Communications Magazine*, 2017, 55(1), pp. 84- 91.

[6] Rahmani, A. M., Gia, T. N., Negash, B., Anzanpour, A., Azimi, I., Jiang, M., Liljeberg, P. Exploiting smart e-Health gateways at the edge of healthcare Internet-of-Things: A fog computing approach, *Future Generation Computer Systems*, 2018, 78, pp. 641-658.

[7] Thibaud, M., Chi, H., Zhou, W., Piramuthu, S., Internet of Things (IoT) in high-risk Environment, Health and Safety (EHS) industries: A comprehensive review, *Decision Support Systems,* 2018, 108, pp. 79-95.

[8] Ayón, C. Unpacking Immigrant Health: Policy, Stress, and Demographics, *Race and Social Problems,* 2018, pp.1-3.

[9] Chaudhary, R., Jindal, A., Aujla, G. S., Kumar, N., Das, A. K., Saxena, N. LSCSH: Lattice-Based Secure Cryptosystem for Smart Healthcare in Smart Cities Environment, *IEEE Communications Magazine,* 2018, 56(4), pp. 24-32.

[10] Abdullah, A., Ismael, A., Rashid, A., Abou-ElNour, A., Tarique, M. Real time wireless health monitoring application using mobile devices, *International Journal of Computer Networks & Communications,* 2015, 7(3), pp. 13-30.

[11] Kakria, P., Tripathi, N. K., Kitipawang, P. A real-time health monitoring system for remote cardiac patients using smartphone and wearable sensors, *International journal of telemedicine and applications*, 2015, 8.

[12] Goldberger, A. L., Amaral, L. A., Hausdorff, J. M., Ivanov, P. C., Peng, C. K., Stanley, H. E. Fractal dynamics in physiology: alterations with disease and aging, *Proceedings of the national academy of sciences,* 2002, 99(1), pp. 2466-2472.

[13] Majumder, S., Mondal, T., Deen, M. J. Wearable sensors for remote health monitoring, *Sensors,* 2017, 17(1), pp. 130.

[14] Saha, J., Saha, A. K., Chatterjee, A., Agrawal, S., Saha, A., Kar, A., Saha, H. N., Advanced IoT based combined remote health monitoring, home automation and alarm system, In *Computing and Communication Workshop and Conference, IEEE 8th Annual, 2018*, pp 602-606.

[15] Kalid, N., Zaidan, A. A., Zaidan, B. B., Salman, O. H., Hashim, M., Muzammil, H. Based Real Time Remote Health Monitoring Systems: A Review on Patients Prioritization and Related "Big Data" Using Body Sensors information and Communication Technology, *Journal of medical systems*, 2018,42(2), pp. 30.

[16] Walinjkar, A., Woods, J. Personalized wearable systems for real-time ECG classification and healthcare interoperability: Realtime ECG classification and FHIR interoperability, In *Internet Technologies and Applications*, 2017, pp. 9-14.

[17] Patel, S., Park, H., Bonato, P., Chan, L., Rodgers, M. A review of wearable sensors and systems with application in rehabilitation, *Journal of neuro engineering and rehabilitation*, 2012, 9(1), pp. 21.

[18] Yang, Z., Zhou, Q., Lei, L., Zheng, K., Xiang, W. An IoT-cloud based wearable ECG monitoring system for smart healthcare, *Journal of medical systems,* 2016, 40(12), pp. 286.

In: Intelligent Information Retrieval … ISBN: 978-1-68507-301-5
Editors: Parma Nand et al. © 2021 Nova Science Publishers, Inc.

Chapter 6

IoT in Healthcare – Applications, Benefits, Challenges, Real-Time Uses, and Cases

Gaddam Prathik Kumar[1], Kanishka Negi[1], Huzaif Muataq Naikoo[1], Subrata Sahana[1,*] and Sanjoy Das[2]

[1]School of Engineering and Technology,
Sharda University, Greater Noida, Uttar Pradesh, India
[2]Indira Gandhi National Tribal University, India

Abstract

Today's healthcare facilities and growing technologies dispense a variety of difficulties to systems, implementers, and designers. IoT is also increasing its effectiveness in every field of healthcare so that it is easier for both patient and doctor to get their works without in a medical environment. However, despite the obstacles, there's a channel running that supports the service providers for their work through the systems and products as the number of people who are in the need of assistance is growing significantly. We present a designed approach in

* Corresponding Author's E-mail: subrata.sahana@gmail.com.

this chapter for elaborating IoT for health care programs. The approach will be demonstrated for use cases, and the quality issues which need to be carefully handled will be discussed. In this chapter, we have discussed different architectures and quality requirements that are essential for IoT applications. We have illustrated and included three of the best use cases of the healthcare field and discussed its quality requirements. We also addressed the need as well as uses of IoT in healthcare, review of different works has done in the research field along with a proposed model or methodology is been compiled and discussed.

Keywords: Internet of Things (IoT), Healthcare, Sensors, IoT Devices Tracking, Privacy

INTRODUCTION

Internet of Things

The Internet impacts a lot of aspects of our daily life. Internet of Things is an upcoming, powerful domain wherein devices work taking help through the internet using sensors, microcontrollers, and transceivers to empower communication. It is a computing method that is constructed using a particular communication stack that permits us to communicate among such devices and operate with the users and turn into a constitutional part of the web as described in Figure 1.

IoT (Internet of Things) has unfolded wide and has been applied in totally different environments including homes, health care institutions, and numerous transportations dominant systems and IoT combinations are some of the most common issues for researchers. Different tactics have been planned to manage IoT devices. IoT security has high priority issues and is the primary topic for research within the field of IoT. Data protection could be a crucial issue for network devices. In the field of IoT, security plays a significant role whenever an attack or interference with IoT devices can cause a threat to human life, particularly with crucial IoT applications (Perrier 2015).

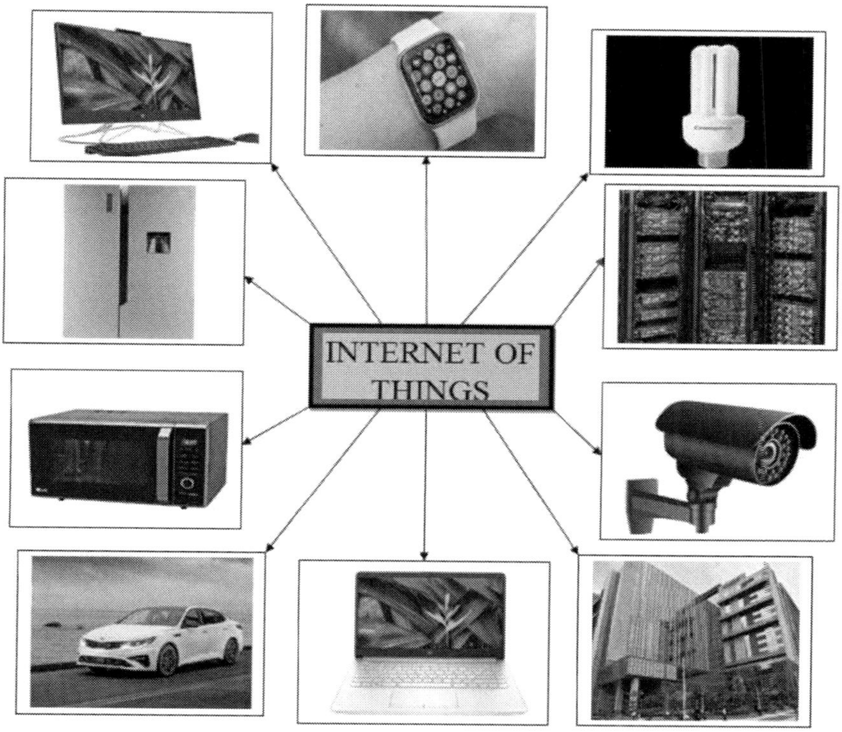

Figure 1. Internet of Things (Atzori, Iera, and Morabito 2010).

Need of IoT Technology in Healthcare

IoT has undoubtedly modified the healthcare industry and has become the most promising communication paradigm. It has redefined the area of devices and how people interact while providing solutions in the healthcare department. IoT has a variety of functions in healthcare that not just provide help to patients but also their families, physicians, hospitals, and insurance companies. It can help us to increase the productivity of various medical applications which can cause a huge impact on the healthcare system in a positive way (Chouffani 2016).

One of the most required and basic needs is healthcare that is required by every person. This results in new and fascinating outcomes and provides a sense of fulfillment thus making the healthcare system gainful or profitable. The goal of the health policy is to improve cost-effectiveness without compromising quality treatment and care as in Figure 2.

However, doctors aren't completely sure about patients in the field of cash and in the field of caring. Another drawback related to the health network is the absence of medical advantages for tracing the medical past of patients. A few years back, a valuation in India was conducted for monitoring the efficient functioning of medical provisions. It was revealed that the patient medical history in many hospitals was not managed properly. Hence, it is essential to improve the healthcare system to make it better (Koppar and Sridhar 2009).

Medical facilities can be optimized with the help of IoT by the means of Electronic Health Record (EHR) in Figure 3 which tracks the patient's medical records to provide them with the applicable treatment or by remote monitoring and communication to keep track of patients as shown in Figure 3.

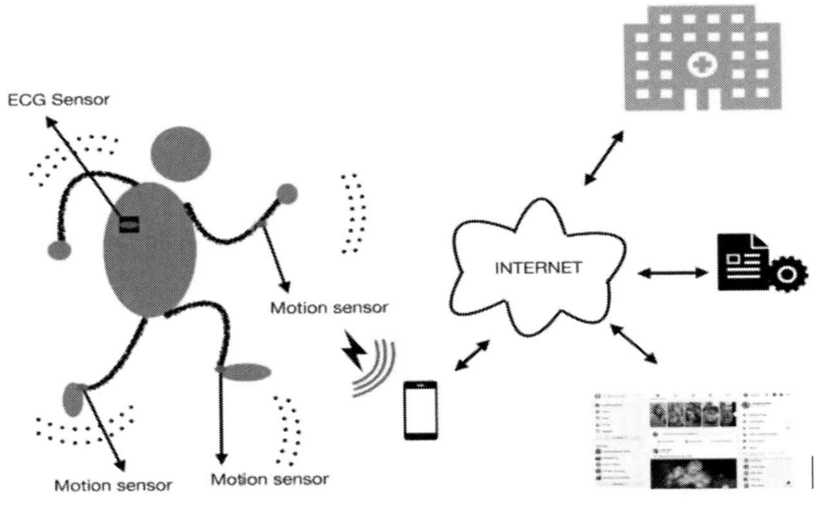

Figure 2. Sensor(Atzori, Iera, and Morabito 2010).

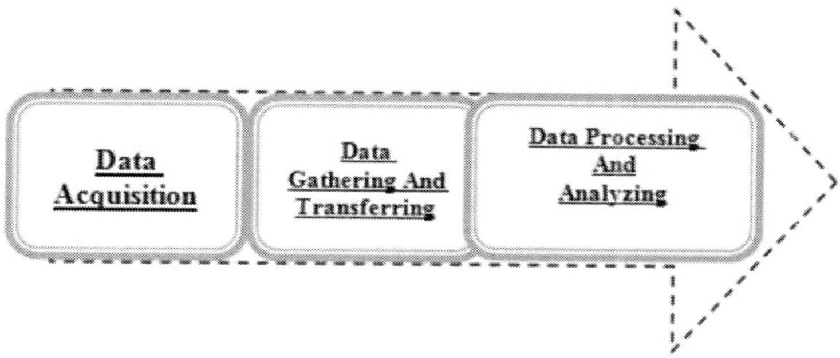

Figure 3. Electronic Health Record Architecture (u Farooq et al. 2015).

IoT can help health care services by maintaining digital identity for every patient, It is useful in observing and analyzing the patient information it simply gathers the information and efficient data that has to be orstored in the cloud network, and then this data can be used during the time of emergency. Knowing any of the medical histories of the patient allows a person to take steps to reduce his or her risk.

Obtuse but inevitably the healthcare industry landscape is changing – and in a positive direction. This massive advancement in technology permits continuous and present medical device access from any connected device over the net. (u Farooq et al. 2015).

An Analysis of the Internet of Things in the Healthcare Environment

Healthcare changes dramatically because of technological developments and the technologies we used in home health are currently improving this by reminding the medicine schedule, remote monitoring, and adding up patients with new medicine data by prescribers through the web. The practice of medicine has been revolutionized by digital technology.

The ongoing SARS-CoV-2COVID-19 pandemic has placed an extraordinary demand on the growth of the modern healthcare system. With this we can view the changes in the upcoming years of the healthcare department the quick response of the industry has demonstrated its adaptability, durability, and the ability to change the system for the better in a short amount of time. We can notice the remarkable change in the healthcare industry. The healthcare sector has produced exceptional examples of innovation and its modernization since the pandemic has started.

The use of technology in healthcare is constantly improving and streamlining the functioning of the healthcare system. With the help of smart technologies consumer can manage their health. For example, an asthma is a measuring device of peak expiratory flow (PEF) this device can help the patient manage their respiratory profile, this can be quickly accessed by the patient if something goes wrong another smart technology is an Insulin pen people with diabetes use this to inject insulin. These technologies are in the hands of consumers. This won't help them for longer periods but for sure can help them in emergencies (Kang, Kim, and Koh 2016).

> "Our task at the moment is to face our fears about the future with courage; to turn to technologies with an open mind and to prepare for the changing world with as much knowledge as possible."

Before the Internet of Things, Maintaining a record of patient medical history was a difficult task and also the patients' interaction with doctors was limited. Now it can be done virtually with the help of IoT. Doctors can keep a check on their patient's health with the help of a remote monitoring system. With the help of IoT applications patients can also keep a check on their health for example: wearing a health watch can detect the signs of atrial fibrillation. And warn you if you should consult a doctor (Ge et al. 2016).

Apart from monitoring patients' health, IoT-based applications are most helpful in hospitals and medical institutions. For example, IoT-based smart wheelchairs with IoV (Yadav et al. 2018)are used for patients tracking with disabilities and helping them to move from one place to another with the help of sensors, provided the obstacle detection system reduces the chance of collision. With the ongoing pandemic, sanitizing hands at regular intervals can prevent the spread of diseases. Devices which are used for hygiene monitoring using IoT- networks IoT-enabled Hygiene monitoring devices are useful in reducing the spread of infection from infectious persons. Various Internet of Things equipments can also be useful in the management of assets like controlling inventory of pharmacy, and monitoring of the environment.

Internet of Things works as an important role in our everyday life. A vast number of such appliances have found their way into our homes, the health and transport industry, and small or even large businesses. But this thriving industry has a major drawback that is device security. Naturally, security measures have been undertaken to shield information, but there is always a risk of hackers breaking into the system and stealing confidential information. The data provided to IoT devices are personal and can be highly sensitive, thus giving rise to an alarming concern about data security.

EFFECTIVENESS OF HEALTHCARE BASED ON IOT AND APPLICATIONS

IoT that is the Internet of Things is evolving in the field of healthcare at an inflating pace over time. It varies from the healthcare industry to personal healthcare and healthcare payment options. At the same time, we see how IoT is growing and how its reality and originality of joined healthcare is accelerating and its real use cases are evolving and catching speed in productivity even if any difficulties come in between.

Many improvements are done with the help of IoT in the fields of medical Science. Most IoT initiative helps in improving the care required for the patient with the help of monitoring through remote and observing. Both this technology help us in tracking the patient's condition and health, if any changes within limits of the pulse rate or respiratory rate are noticed, an instant alert message is sent to the physician informing him/her that the threshold value has been breached. The growth and development of IoT showed the potential and capacity to transform modern healthcare positively. Health data is sensitive as it contains all the information about the patient if it would be misused then it can cause damage to the privacy of people.

Applications

IoT Application could be the next frontier in the race of its share of the wallet. Application with IoT has superior sensors and revolutionary computing capabilities which are proven a boon for the healthcare industry.

RemotePatient Monitoring

Visiting hospitals for regular check-ups is surely the least favorite activity in society.RPM (Remote Patient Monitoring) is a device that helps us to manage patient health virtually. As technology is improving day by day this device can gather patients outside of traditional healthcare settings. RPM can indirectly help physicians also as it increases the capacity for physicians to treat more patients. The patient is continuously monitored, and accordingly, physicians suggest solutions for the patient virtually. Also, RPM can reduce the risk of infection, People who are facing acute or chronic diseases such as cardiovascular disease or preterm birth can avoid unnecessary trips to clinics and this decreases their risk of contact with patients and prevents them from the risk of infection. The patient is continuously monitored; accordingly, physicians suggest solutions for the patient. In Figure 4 it shows how Remote Patient Monitoring works as Figure 4 (Holler et al. 2014).

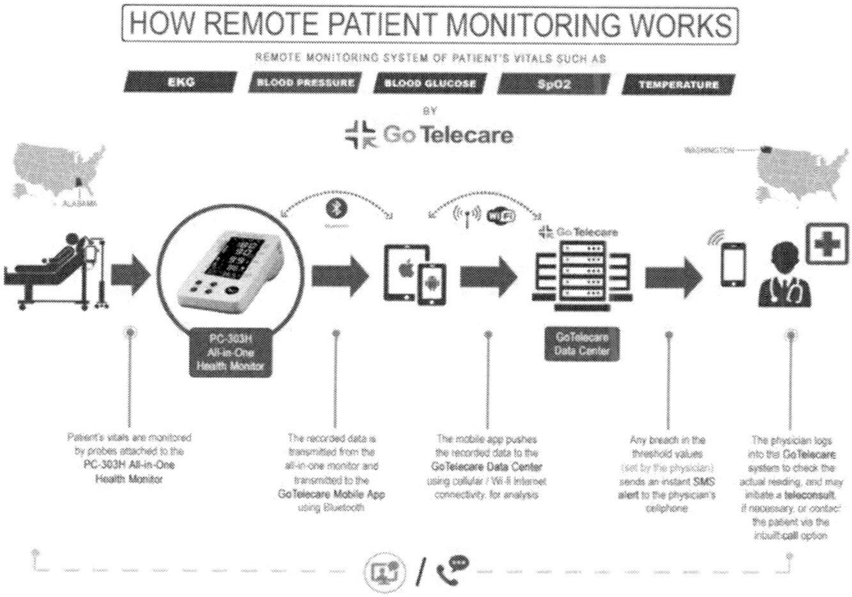

Figure 4.Working of Remote Patient Monitoring.

Wearable Healthcare Device

Wearable healthcare devices are one of the most impactful applications in today's world. In n the United States of America the use of wearable healthcare devices went from 9% in 2014 to 33% in 2018, the improvement in such devices and their surging demand has influenced and revolutionized the medical industry. By improving efficiency and lowering the operational costs and helping the providers offer a better standard of care through this, the healthcare industry had caught up on healthcare wearables very soon. Wearable application has superior sensors which help has to detect pulses at an emergency such as cardiac arrest, vasovagal syncope as Figure 5. Another use of the wearable application is for taking note of respiratory rate i.e. the number of breaths a patient takes per minute. It could help us aid in the identification of asthma attacks beforehand. And it can also be used to detect fever, heatstroke (Pointer 2014).

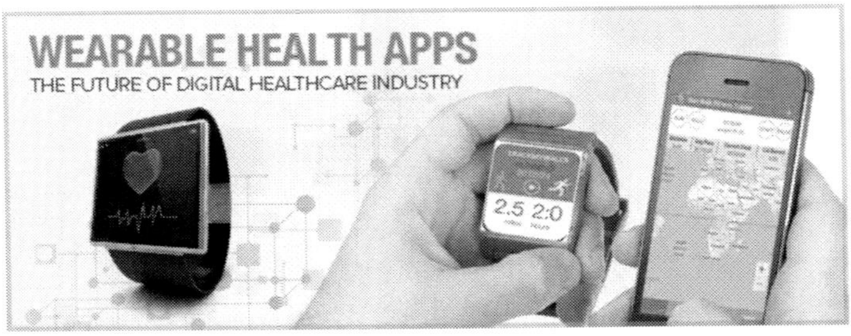

Figure 5. Wearable Device.

Hand Hygiene Monitoring

As we know that we are facing this global pandemic COVID-19 and one of the most important things to protect yourself from COVID is to wear a mask and sanitize your hand regularly to minimize the risk of spreading contagion. Today many hospitals, offices educational institutes use IOT build no-touch hand sanitizer dispensers. For any press-to-release hand sanitizer, we have a contactless hand sanitizer dispenser. The servo motor is instructed by the Arduino to actuate and dispense the sanitizer as soon as a hand of the person is placed below the hygiene sanitizer and a person's hand comes below the sanitizer and hinder the line of the sight of the sensors embedded in it. These devices remind people to sanitize their hands when they enter any of the premises. The device can give instructions on how to sanitize to mitigate a particular risk for a particular person as Figure 6.

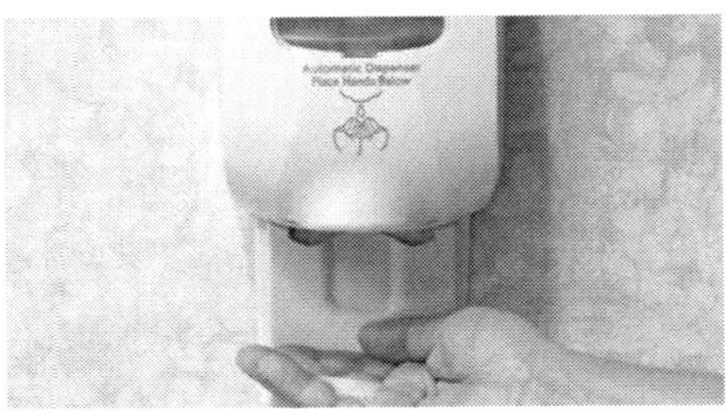

Figure 6. Sanitizer Spray Machine.

Smart Wheelchair

An IoT-based smart wheelchair works on the sensor and associative technology. It is built around a matched pair of transducers that convert movement into electrical energy and vice versa. A proper working smart chair with full automation is a boon for disabled people. Fully automatic wheelchairs can support disabled people to move freely in home, work, or hospital; it increases the mobility and independence for the user and their carrier as Figure 7. This IoT-based smart wheelchair is also provided with an obstacle detection system that reduces the chance of collision (Pointer 2014).

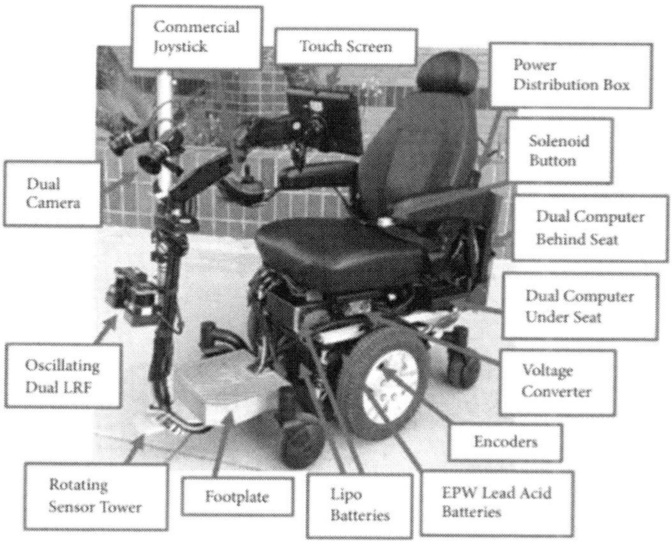

Figure 7. Smart Wheelchair (Soh and Demiris 2015).

IoT Architecture for Healthcare Networks

IoT-based architecture of healthcare systems has developed in recent years. The following are amply elaborated healthcare systems.

mHEALTH

Intending to bring IoT is effective action in healthcare, structured support is required which connects the IoT sensors to whole health care systems, that is mHealth (Almotiri, Khan, and Alghamdi 2016). Is an efficient example of it. It's a hierarchical architecture as shown in Figure 8 below. The first section is the Data collection which incorporates IoT devices used for nirecognizing and for collecting and saving the health-specific parameters. A blood sugar sensing device, ECG test devices, etc are some of the examples. The second section is Data storage takes the charge of storing the health data cleanly and clearly. Third and the final section is the Data processing layer which examines the sensor data. It uses non-artificial intelligence and artificial intelligence-based techniques as Figure 8.

The sensors will transfer the technical data to the last two sections (the layer of storing data& the layer of processing the data). The technology of mHealth can be used with ANT, Bluetooth, Zigbee, and NFC or WiFi.

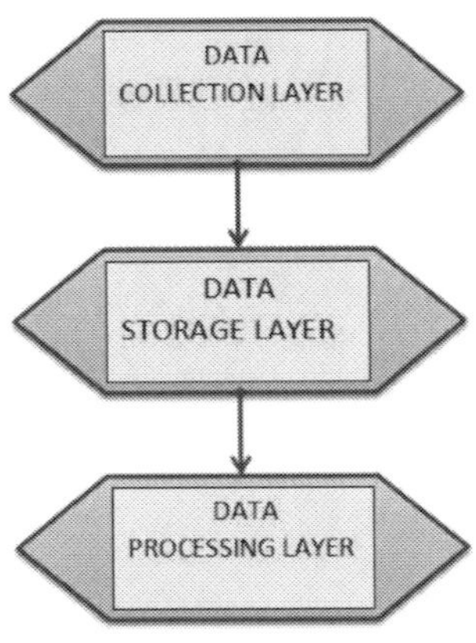

Figure 8. mHealth end-to-end architecture system(Kumar 2017).

Protocol Based on Constrained Application Architecture

(CoAP) Constrained Application System(Shelby and Bormann 2011; Ugrenovic and Gardasevic 2015) is an execution layer system framed for the devices andtypes of equipment that are based on constrained, for example – Sensors(Khattak, Ruta, and Di Sciascio 2014). CoAP working working isbased on the REST paradigm which is also known as Representational State Transfer. Table1 below shows the healthcare protocol stack based on the CoAP stack(Ugrenovic and Gardasevic 2015).

Table 1. CoAP System stack for the healthcare networks (Kumar 2017)

Traditional Stack	CoAP Stack
Layer of Application	Based on CoAP
Layer of transport	Based on UDP
Layer of Network	Based on IPV6/RPL
A layer of Network Adaption	Based on 6LoWPAN
A layer of Datalink	Works on 802.15.4
Physical layer	Works on 802.15.4

Protocol which is CoAP based maintains the communication by making it reliable (Confirmedas well as Acknowledged messages are used) and the best effort communication (NON-message is used). Any one of the techniques can be used by Healthcare systems that use CoAP for transferring the data collected by sensors to the suitable. HTTP and the networks based on CoAP are similar to a large extent. These two protocols work or follows 4 basic techniques and commands to transfer the data collected by sensors that are DELETE, PUT, GET, and at last POST.

6LoWPAN Healthcare Architecture System

Now - a - days internet protocols i.e., IP networks are everywhere. Thus, the healthcare system uses the networks of IP for transferring the data of IoT. But, the networks of IPV-6requires a huge weightage of bandwidth and compiling energy. Therefore, we look for unfaltering network coverage which is not permissible in the case of IoT devices. Thus, healthcare architectures preferred 6LoWPAN over IP networks (Shelby and Bormann 2011). The sensor nodes use the 6LoWPAN network stack to transfer data to the network. The 6LoWPAN is used by health sensors with an end-to-end network. The data collected by sensors is introduced inside the datagram based on 6LoWPAN & passed on into the IEEE802.15.4 network tothe gateway or the router which is present at the ending or the edge(Gia et al. 2014). After that, the IPV6 protocol packets are transfigured by the network gateway, then transfers to traditional IPV6 networks for further compiling of data.

Standard Health Architecture Based on IEEE 11073

The IEEE 11073 has been introduced by the IEEE 11073 health standard (Kang, Kim, and Koh 2016) which is especially being introduced for fitness devices and personal health. For instance, medication dispenses glucose level monitors, activity monitors, etc. The planning reached out to the network through one extra more layer ofIEEEnetwork which is based on IEEE 110073. One of the main feature that is used by the architecture that is proposed is the usage of the DTLS which is also known as Datagram Transport layer security. This is known by all that the protocol network known as UDP is not encrypted by any technique. Although Data related to Health is required to protect it from malicious attacks & eavesdropping. Consequently, the architecture that is proposed applied an additional secured layer on top of the UDP protocol.

The 6LOWPAN network protocol is been used to liaise in accordance with the server of healthcare. Then, a data back transmitted transformed into theIPV4/V6 & then this thing is transferred to the client of the web using the HTTP for the data compilation. Healthcare professionals and doctors then use the web client to track the health of the patients. DIM (Kang, Kim, and Koh 2016) (Domain Information Model) is been defined as the exchange of messages which are related to healthcare with the help of IEEE 11073 system-based protocol(Ge et al. 2016).DIM simply provides overall domain like research done clinically, nursing, and healthcare field. This DIM is usually created to present the semantics of an overall domain with the help of languages in which subject matters understand by experts using some UML classical diagrams. Through this model, it can show the concept like domain activities, places, and people also, at last, it shows how every concept is related to one another in the DIMs.

Use Cases General Categorisation for IoT Based Healthcare System

Healthcare is generally classified into 3wide-field case types:

1. Long-term case
2. Acute case
3. Community-based case

Long Term Case

Long-term cases are introduced to skilled nursing facilities or nursing homes, where patients reside for years, months, or weeks and where the caretakers are paid, professionals.

Acute Case

Caretaker is paid healthcare professional

Community-Based Case

Caretakers take care of the patients at their own houses and paid professional or unpaid members of the family or friends. For collecting data IOT's protocols are used for those surroundings and then the data are piled by the usage of analytics and after that, the information reports to the caretakers. Under this, we have three classes or categories of real-world use cases of healthcare such as:

- Human tracking or tracking of the humans
- Things tracking or tracking of the things
- Tracking Humans and Things.

Human Tracking or Tracking of the Humans

These are the Class A systems that imply tracking human data. For example --- Caretakers, Patients, Family members by the use of IoT devices. Maybe this is a widely developed area in healthcare in the broad area of IoT(Internet ofThings) is patients data--gathering. At Present, telemetry monitors are used to monitor or transfer temperature of the body, BP, urine output, EKG stats, and so on, whereas EKG simply means electrocardiography in which it records the signals that are electrical from our hearts for the checking of various heart conditions. Through analyzing the crucial signs, the expert people can easily be detected and start caring beforehand for diseases like - Heart failure, cancer, or any infectious disease. Other examples also can be given under this class which includes physical spot identification or tracking the site of the victims in many areas of the settings (Home/House, Long-termed, or Acute).

The victims are added to the ER system for tracking and identifying the person(DISEASED PATIENT) who is having dementia, the victims having a disease called Alzheimer's, or one with behavior which self-destroying like cutting suicidal behavior or bulimia could be easily geo-located or identified by IoT. These tracking can initially be compiled or implemented with the help of GPS bracelets systems, but the sensors that are proximity sensors connected with the help of the internet or technologies which are based on cloud systems could permit tracking the entities inner of the facilities like homes, or out of the houses that are an outside environment where signals of the GPS may be difficult to reach. This IoT device is very useful for Healthcare systems that provide operating in areas that are at high risk. E.g., like Caring about mental-health that might give advantages from tracing for security causes.

Things Trackings or Tracking of Things

These are Class B which includes the things tracking or identification in a real-world-time health care setting. It could include supplies, medical device specimens, and so on. For instance, In case of an emergency, certain shared equipment availability is short (for example--intermittent pressure devices, EKG machines, intravenous pumps). Examples like the Airfinder is a system that locates things in real-time uses a technology called symphony link which tracks and analyzes the supplies into a whole hospital or facilities and also into the operating room(Laplante et al. 2017).

Hospital staff and Nurses might in some situation keep the materials or equipment with them due to which those types of equipment can be accessed by the nurses when it required, somehow a problem can be created if the other ward is also in the requirement of the same equipment but he is unable to locate it due to non-availability. In such conditions, these IoT devices could be a lifesaver. IoT can help in identifying or tracking and requirement for the supplies replacement. Most of the equipment has this alarm feature for numerous deviation.

For Example-- Refill, Failure, Time to calibrate readings exceed, and so on. Recurring tools alarms can cause staff and nurses to become aware of the alarming fatigue so that their reaction is not brisk enough for handling an exceptional situation. Different kinds of alarms could be set up for difficult situations& transfers the signs of alarms to the relevant healthcare professionals.

Tracking the Things and Humans

Here the title 'tracking things and human' is been applied as class C which involves a hybrid of class A which is (Human Tracking) and Class B that is (Things Tracking). The IoT application categoriesgive9 general and dimensions of care settings use cases that are: (Chouffani 2016)

- Long term (A class, B class, C class)
- Home (A class, B class, C class)
- Acute (A class, B class, C class)

Real-World Use Case For IoT in Health Care

The healthcare's general framework describes the IoT applications by considering the following three of the use cases:

1. Victim having Alzheimer's disease.
2. Victim or the staff security issues or concerns in hospital settings.
3. Victim having alcohol habituation.

Here we have described a scenario that forms a health-checking provider's perspective through the usage of the frameworks set--up, Implying how an IoT could help in patient care and in monitoring.

Use Case of Alcohol-Habituation

This is a chronic disease that remains for the long term, In this disease, a victim develops a habit of consuming alcohol at a high level. In the early phases of the therapy, a victim might tolerate AWS that is (Alcoholic withdrawal syndrome). For example, in the USA about 14 million people are either a lot addicted to alcohol or abusers after drinking alcohol. In such cases the victim may go through the following physical and emotional symptoms (Laplante 2017):

1. headache
2. Loss Of appetite
3. Insomnia
4. Shakiness
5. Depression
6. Sweating
7. Anxiety
8. Irritability
9. Fatigue
10. Vomiting or nausea

Table 2. AWS Use Case Construct [23]

MODEL ELEMENT REALIZATION		
1.	SENSOR	Proximity Sensor
2.	SNAPSHOT(TIME)	Once Per Minute 3.
3.	CLUSTER	Set of (3) Proximity Sensors.
4.	AGGREGATOR	Determine severity of AWS symptom.
5.	COMMUNICATION	ZigBee1 compliant network of Sensor wired (Internet) to eUtility.
6.	e UTILITY	Remote monitoring software.
7.	DECISION	Degree of existing AWS symptoms.

AWS symptoms could conclusively be monitored by using (non-internet-enabled analytics) or theNoT system. For example like Victim with AWS needs to take care appropriately regarding irregular movements and trembling. The sensor could be placed deliberately in the victim's house to keep him on track by monitoring slight changes in its activities like - bathroom usage via an IoT. The sensor can also detect the odor of the vomit which provides extra uses in the treatment and care of the AWS victim in HOME-care system settings.

Victim's Having Alzheimer's Disease

The most common form of mental illness is Alzheimer's Disease, which reaches 60-80% of overall cases[12]. Reports have shown that 1 in 9 people who are at the age of sixty-five years and those who are older than 65 have this disease called Alzheimer's.

Patients having Alzheimer's disease may have the following symptoms:

1. Difficulty in speaking or writing the words.
2. Trouble understanding spatial relationships and visual images.
3. Confusion with place or time.
4. Faces problems completing simple tasks at home or the workplace.
5. Loss of memory creates confusion.

Table 3. Alzheimer's Use Case Construct [23]

MODEL ELEMENT		REALIZATION
1.	SENSOR	Proximity Sensor(s)
2.	SNAPSHOT(TIME)	Every 30 s.
3.	CLUSTER	Set of (3) Proximity Sensors Per room
4.	AGGREGATOR	Determine Location.
5.	WEIGHT	Room layout dependent.
6.	COMMUNICATION	WiFi network of sensors or clusters or wired (internet) to eUtility.
7.	e UTILITY	Remote monitoring software.
8.	DECISION	Patient wandering or patient not Wandering ,dispatch assistance.

Some of those signs of symptoms can be conclusively analyzed through using IoT devices and it also monitors. As the disease makes progress in an individual. The functional abilities and cognitive ability can decline. When the victims deal with the difficulty of moving here and there, then it is obvious that they having pneumonia and infection which is at higher risk, due to which it often causes the patient to die those who have Alzheimer's disease. Thus, the toll is taken by this disease on caregivers and patients, where there is a requirement to that such automation which can help the caregivers at a wide area of stages of Alzheimer's. Victims who are having Alzheimer's disease require focus care of the best quality. Mainly in the initial phases, the victim's level of freedom.

Thus, the healthcare providers and caregivers must provide safety to the victim unless harming its independence. Here, IoT devices could be lifesaver devices like- Radiofrequency (RFID) chips that could be placed on the patient's clothing for easier tracking and them to feel that they are being watched.

The patient's movement and position can be tracked by the sensors. Caregivers could be notified in case of an emergency. If the patient gets upset, the machines that are sensors can automatically be ready to identify/detects/track the blood pressure and heartbeat. If the victim's daziness is increasing more and becoming more wandering, then the sensor can track the required pattern which is wandering, and detects it. One of the drawbacks here is privacy. However, information about the patient is conclusively been revealing outwards of the immediate caregivers.

Use Cases of Safety and Patient

There are some very important issues, those are violence and safety. Also, large numbers of outbreaks of violence that are horizontal like visitors and family outbreaks of violence against the healthcare providers and also nurses fought against nurses.

Institutions of health care are provided with full security video surveillance networks, but the thing is that if devices like metal detectors are also included in institutions with an efficient IOT technology cloud system then it can provide additional safety against violence with dangerous weapons like knives, guns, etc.

Providers of the health care systems debated on these issues of metal detectors and some of them believed that the unsafe of the metal detectors are against the culture or the practices of the severe care surroundings and environment because they recognized as the equipment of the prison. On the other hand, some of them have taken this situation as a future for the healthcare institution and supported the use of metal detectors in the health care systems in institutions [23].

Table 4. Safety Use Case Construct [23]

MODEL ELEMENT		REALIZATION
1.	SENSOR	Proximity Sensor
2.	SNAPSHOT(TIME)	Based on Need.
3.	CLUSTER	Set of (3) Proximity Sensors.
4.	AGGREGATOR	Determine Aggressive Behaviour.
5.	COMMUNICATION	Bluetooth network of Sensor wired (Internet) to eUtility.
6.	e UTILITY	Remote monitoring software.
7.	DECISION	Patient or staff in danger or patient staff not in danger, dispatch assistance

Requirements of Quality for IoT in Healthcare Applications

When the purpose of IoT healthcare applications is stated, light is always focused on the following concerns; fitness purposes, wireless interoperability, the efficiency of the energy, and so on (Laplante 2017). As of now, IoT is being used in every aspect of life however there is a majority of concern that is regarding the requirement of quality. 3 explicit qualities necessities (security need, need of patient safety, and caring requirement, mainly) in the healthcare system applications are mainly of special and crucial importance due to the information's nature which is personal and sensitive.

Requirements for the Privacy

The crucial aspect of healthcare is the privacy of patients. People always expect their personally identifiable information will remain safe with the healthcare providers. Privacy assurance must be given by IoT healthcare systems, however, it must allow sharing of details when it is extremely needed (McCue 2015).

The HIPAA Act defines how a patient's details and health information should be shared and used to maintain privacy while allowing the patient to share the details when needed to provide elite care. HIPAA has an integral role in healthcare. However, new queries have come up about the relationship between IoT and HIPAA.

A new report reported privacy legislation on the built-in security of IoT devices, security breaches, and data minimization [15]. Canada's headquarters of privacy commissioner provided a report of 34 pages [16] in February 2016, in which it indicates the concerns for the privacy and information because IoT is continuing to take the position or shape: The reports state that the "IoT has being contrasted with the planet'snervous system or the electricity, for illustrating phenomena which are at unseen, pervasion at once and also will be becoming an importantly unified within the society's fabric "(Morgan 2017)." Many of the worldwide geniuses, thinkers, experts, and builders of technology are providing intense economic social and political conversions, concerns in regarding the surveillance, security, and privacy which are main in between them."

Requirements for the Safety

Safety in the healthcare industry is one of the crucial requirements. These requirements are defined for risk reduction. Medical errors may occur in different healthcare settings, and those that happen in medical areas or hospitals can have harmful consequences. In The USA, the FDAstudy helped us to identify the fault and failure in the system and provide us appropriate solutions to improve the safety of the device. They also found that "known best practices may not be used at all or maybe misused." Wallace and Kuhn said that engineers have to do the below-mentioned points so that the medicals devices that are safe can get generation requirements.

1. collect failure and fault data (from previous and related systems);
2. understand the different types of mistakes that are universal for a specific domain;
3. after collecting information about the fault from prevention and detection approaches certain to these affairs(Laplante et al. 2017).

Requirements for the Caring

An act or a way to approach a patient can be understood as caring. Caring can be an attribute that one owns, and often an adjective to express what is known to be a"good" caregiver. Most nurses will be able to vocalize their notion of caring if questioned. The link between nurses and caring has also been highlighted by Lachman by putting light on that "caring and nursing are so intertwined that nursing always appeared on the same page in a Google search for the definition of caring."

While in the current system where IoT devices have accelerated in every field it has also impacted the healthcare industry(Bergeles and Yang 2013).

In Current systems, IoT embedded robots are being used to mimic the movement of human surgeons, fully autonomous robot surgical systems are envisioned soon that can fully replace surgeons and nurses. However, machines don't have feelings then what should the patient expect in terms of a care system. Caring and related requirements may emerge from laws and regulations, for example, in the robotic surgery system case, HIPAA, The Health Insurance Portability And Accountability act was signed into law in 1996 (Bergeles and Yang 2013). It is legislation to keep patients medical information safe and provide security provisions and data privacy.

RELATED STUDY AND LITERATURE SURVEY

The chapter proposes asecurity model for a health care system to secure medical data transmission in IoT environments. Various security requirements such as authentication, integrity, confidentiality were discussed. The model comprises four continuous processes. It comprises four continuous processes:

1. The data given by the patient is confidential. The data is encrypted using a proposed scheme (cryptographic scheme, which is composed of encryption and decryption processes) and algorithms.
2. Then that encrypted data is being concealed in a cover image using either 2D-DWT-1L or 2D-DWT-2L
3. After data is concealed a Stego image is produced and accordingly the embedded data is extracted. (the 2DDWT-2L technique is carried to extract the secret message and retrieve the cover image)
4. The extracted data is decrypted to retrieve the original data. (Banka, Madan, and Saranya 2018)

In this chapter, an EK-healthcare (Enhanced k-healthcare) model has been explained. Earlier in the chapter, we have seen how the internet can help us to get the details of patients (Name, Age, medical history, medicine, and so on) in this model. A new modal is proposed by enhancing and improving the functionality of the existing research proposed.

When a patient is in an emergency and the doctor is unable to access the internet, he/she still gets to know it by the mobile phone SMS having the information about the patient's emergency. Previously, the data sharing and alerts were through the Internet or K-Healthcare platform but now with the help of this feature, it will be possible for them to get aid through Mobile phone SMS alerts even if they can't access the internet services (Ullah, Shah, and Zhang 2016).

The E-K healthcare modal consist of four-layer as described in Figure 9: (Ullah, Shah, and Zhang 2016)

1. Sensor Layer: This layer consists of body sensors (Arduino & Raspberry pi, oxygen saturation monitoring sensors) and is used to capture the health of a person which can be monitored through wearable devices of mobile phone sensor ex. a heartbeat detector sensor, senses the rate of the heartbeat of a person.
2. Network Layer: Different communication protocols like TCP/IP are used to connect sensor devices with LAN/WAN through this layer. The sensor device sends the information to another device through the network.
3. Mobile/Internet Layer: This layer is used to store data or medical history of a patient and it can be accessed by a physician at the time of emergency directly via mobile or it can be sent to servers through SMS.
4. Services Layer: In this layer, the data is only concerned with the medical staff which can be accessed through any interface.

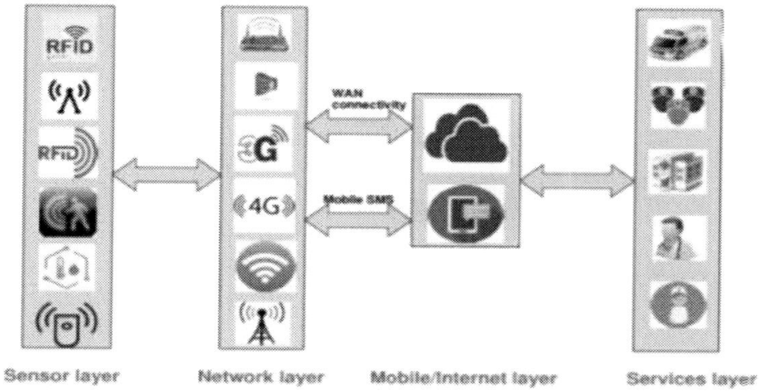

Figure 9. EK-healthcare Model(Ullah, Shah, and Zhang 2016).

Pooja Kanaseand and Sneha Gaikwad in this research chapter have completely changed the components, rather than different sensors that will be needed in smartphones. In the 21st century, smartphones have become an important part of our life isn't it interesting to keep a check of our health through our smartphones now that everything is turning smart? So for a better approach healthcare system has to upgrade itself to a smart system.

The idea shared in this research chapter is that patients will be given smartwatches that keep checking on their health 24/7 till they are admitted to the hospital, the report or data collected will be sent to the doctor for a regular checkup. The smartwatches are further connected to the patient's smartphones or to the patient relatives to keep a check. the major advantage of this system is that anyone can track the patient's help from anyone and also a smartphone is a device that everyone is aware of. (Kassab and Mazzara 2019).

Proposed Model for Healthcare System

In Figure 10, the flow diagram that I mentioned above tells how the information of the health check-up of the patient is retrieved with the help of monitoring different entities and parameters and uses that to identify if the victim or patient is suffering from any of the chronic disorders or other dangerous diseases.

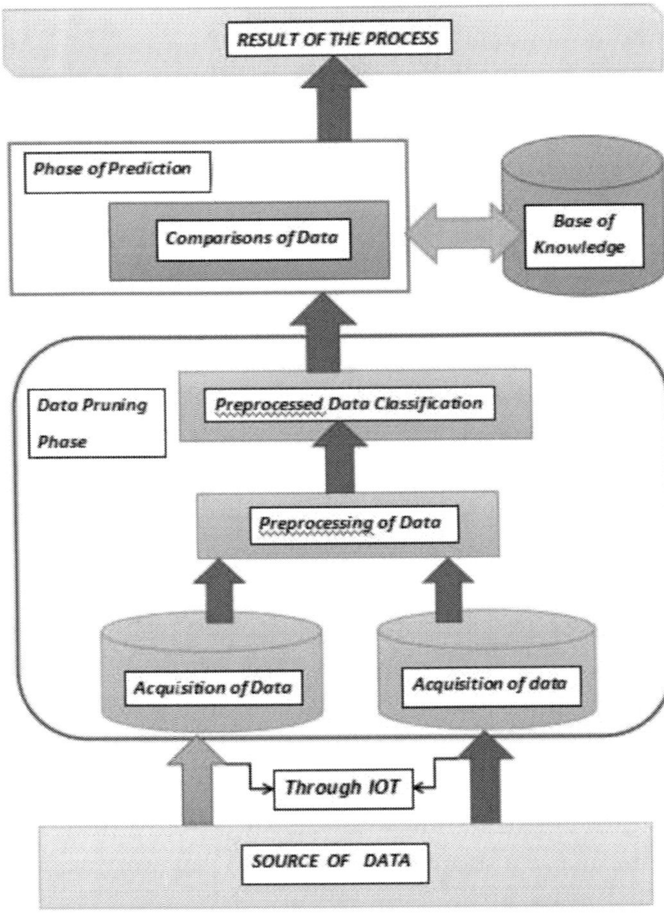

Figure 10. Proposed Model For Iot Based Healthcare System(Banka, Madan, and Saranya 2018).

In tier 1, Different IoT devices collect the various unprocessed data and this information is stored on the cloud server. These IoT devices like sensors that include vibration sensors, pulse sensors, temperature sensors, and BP sensors. some of the devices may give analog output, so to convert it into digital output or signal we have to use the converter IC.

Then using some coding system we read the appropriate values collected by the sensors and then upload or modify them into the database at usual intervals.

In tier 2, By classifying, categorizing, and filtering, we obtain a piece of suitable information as an output result from the stored data. The information is the patient's health care symptoms and data which is in real-time. Now the collected information is transferred to the next level so that we can further predict that if the patient is having any normal or severe kind of disease. By this working of levels its make efficient and smart health care system.

In tier 3, It is the level at which the prediction and analysis take place. The whole system that is designed in which this tier uses data mining techniques to identify the nature and the type of disorders or the disease the patient has. We can use AI technology to improve the overall system by modifying it to be smarter. Therefore, disorder or disease can be deduced by us with the help of the base of knowledge we have right now and we can classify and categorize the output(result) in categories that are different like normal, ideal, and with Symptoms, so on.

Challenges in IoT Based Healthcare System

IoT is used by many various types of applications and gives a great structure for healthcare systems like monitoring of the patient, patient who is diabetic having a smart home system. Many various problems come in between the system of healthcare.

- ECG monitoring uses a supervised manner to analyze and classify the output signals in most cases which increases the cost a lot and during the detection, it can produce errors also. So machine learning can be used to improve the working and efficiency due to which the cost also decreases. This can also use to analyze the signals

- Few of the devices which are worn by the patient for analyzing the healthcare status may be uncomfortable. Since IoT provides the high flexibility that is constant care is required by patient and victim can get the treatment alone from the home instead of visiting the hospitaland can be regularly monitored with the help of internet of things technology
- Another problem is the increase in the leakage of power, high consumption of energy, and the large number of sensors that require high energy for processing. Therefore to reduce this we can use an algorithm that is optimized so that the energy usage can be decreased.
- Data that is transferred from the sensors to the control devices then after that from the control device to the center which monitors the data can be affected due to the noise in between the traveling process. Noise cancellation or removal techniques and efficient architectures can help the data to transfer without altering the nature and also enhance the signals containing data.
- Network Bandwidth with high efficiency is required to read every natural data manufactured by the millions of devices and sensors which are associated.
- Good infrastructure which matches with the large amount of data generated at a high rapidity is required.
- Large storage and the mainframes are required to collect the various patient's or victim's health data which is monitored by the IoT. Cloud can be used to overcome the problem of storage but at the same time, the cloud technology which is used with Integrated IoT can increase the complexity.
- A robust analyzing stage is required at the beginning for effective mining which is cost-effective and meaningful and analyzing the imputed intervals or events.
- Archival of data which is defined, retention, and the purging in the system could increase complexity and its puzzling task for the large quantity of data that is collected which gets caused by the devices like sensors or other equipment.

- Not having consistent standards for the data which is generated through the devices can result in generated data and can also prevent extensive adoption.
- One of the main problems of the IoT is that the privacy factors since the devices in the system are more exposed due to which a cyber attack can occur. It is difficult to apply encryption techniques on devices because the devices are less resource compulsorily.
- Connected devices have lots of risk of hacking due to which system can malfunction due to which there is the potential of security implications. So to reduce its potential security implications authentications and other unique management should be implemented.
- The number of devices that are connected may increase extremely due to which the prerequisite architecture that is to be ascendable or scalable system applications has to have the competencies incorporation along with the wide varieties of the systems and the devices.

DISCUSSION

In this chapter we have discussed what IoT is and how it is revolutionizing our everyday life – IoT is everywhere. We have also mentioned applications, future challenges, and benefits of the internet of things (IoT).IoT promises to drive significant changes and make a huge impact on the healthcare system. This chapter reviews the diverse facet of IoT-based healthcare technologies and the effectiveness of IoT in Healthcare. We have also focused on Quality requirements for IoT in healthcare. Despite the various advantages, IoT faces some challenges. More reliable and better services if these challenges are met and overcome in the field of IoT.

CONCLUSION AND FUTURE SCOPE

In this chapter writing, we have presented the overall and important uses of IoT in the healthcare field the chapter is based on the healthcare division where IoT can be applied. Firstly, we have shown and included the overview of the Internet of Things, its definition and working of IoT in real life, and its need in the healthcare section. After that, we have introduced an overall analysis of healthcare based on IoT and its applications. Then we have provided different architecture of IoT in the healthcare field. Then we have provided a classification for healthcare cases like tracking humans, tracking things, and tracking human & things both. Afterward, we studied different real-world use cases of IoT-based healthcare systems and included them in this chapter. After that, we included the requirements for the best IOT application in health care. Then we have researched the previous works done by different people about how IoT can work in the HEALTH CARE field and their proposed works. Then we have given our simple and understandable proposed model of IoT in the healthcare field. After that, we have introduced some of the challenges coming in between working with IoT in healthcare systems. In the end, we have discussed the chapter that IOT in the broader field and its uses in a brief way related to our chapter writing that how the IoT is going to be an essential sector in the healthcare field.

By reading this chapter writing anyone can easily understand due to its simple and understandable concepts and words. Its main aim is to connect or bind the earlier generation, present as well as future generations so that generations can connect themselves that how IoT is increasing in different fields of life. Basically through this chapter, the urban areas, as well as rural areas, can also be developed by introducing a strong base of IoT. In the future, the proposed systems can also be set up in the hospital's clinics of urban and rural areas, and so that a large amount of data can be acquired which is stored in an online cloud or database. These data can be accessed from a smart mobile through a special application. In rural areas, those patients who can able to move to urban areas for better medical assistance by the doctor can also get assisted and cured easily by a doctor who is at a large distance with the help of INTERNET OF THINGS. Finally, IoT is also provided security of the system in healthcare so the patient can remain tension-free so that its medical assistance can be disturbed. IoT is the future of the different real world works in different fields which makes our works easier and comfortable to handle.

References

Almotiri, Sultan H, Murtaza A Khan, and Mohammed A Alghamdi. 2016. "Mobile Health (m-Health) System in the Context of IoT." In *2016 IEEE 4th International Conference on Future Internet of Things and Cloud Workshops (FiCloudW)*, 39–42.

Atzori, Luigi, Antonio Iera, and Giacomo Morabito. 2010. "The Internet of Things: A Survey."*Computer Networks* 54 (15): 2787–2805.

Banka, Shubham, Isha Madan, and S S Saranya. 2018. "Smart Healthcare Monitoring Using IoT."*International Journal of Applied Engineering Research* 13 (15): 11984–89.

Bergeles, Christos, and Guang-Zhong Yang. 2013. "From Passive Tool Holders to Microsurgeons: Safer, Smaller, Smarter Surgical Robots."*IEEE Transactions on Biomedical Engineering* 61 (5): 1565–76.

Chouffani, Reda. 2016. *Can We Expect the Internet of Things in Healthcare.*

Ge, Shu-yuan, Seung-Man Chun, Hyun-Su Kim, and Jong-Tae Park. 2016. "Design and Implementation of Interoperable IoT Healthcare System Based on International Standards." In *2016 13th IEEE Annual Consumer Communications & Networking Conference (CCNC)*, 119–24.

Gia, Tuan Nguyen, Nanda Kumar Thanigaivelan, Amir-Mohammad Rahmani, Tomi Westerlund, Pasi Liljeberg, and Hannu Tenhunen. 2014. "Customizing 6LoWPAN Networks towards Internet-of-

Things Based Ubiquitous Healthcare Systems." In *2014 NORCHIP*, 1–6.

Holler, Jan, Vlasios Tsiatsis, Catherine Mulligan, Stamatis Karnouskos, Stefan Avesand, and David Boyle. 2014. *Internet of Things*. Academic Press.

Kang, Hyung-Woo, Cheol-Min Kim, and Seok-Joo Koh. 2016. "ISO/IEEE 11073-Based Healthcare Services over IoT Platform Using 6LoWPAN and BLE: Architecture and Experimentation." In *2016 International Conference on Networking and Network Applications (NaNA)*, 313–18.

Kassab, Mohamad, and Manuel Mazzara. 2019. "Towards Designing Smart Learning Environments with IoT." In *International Workshop on Software Engineering Aspects of Continuous Development and New Paradigms of Software Production and Deployment*, 152–66.

Khattak, Hasan Ali, Michele Ruta, and Eugenio Eugenio Di Sciascio. 2014. "CoAP-Based Healthcare Sensor Networks: A Survey." In *Proceedings of 2014 11th International Bhurban Conference on Applied Sciences & Technology (IBCAST) Islamabad, Pakistan, 14th-18th January 2014*, 499–503.

Koppar, Anant R, and Venugopalachar Sridhar. 2009. "A Workflow Solution for Electronic Health Records to Improve Healthcare Delivery Efficiency in Rural India." In *2009 International Conference on EHealth, Telemedicine, and Social Medicine*, 227–32.

Kumar, Niharika. 2017. "IoT Architecture and System Design for Healthcare Systems." In *2017 International Conference on Smart Technologies for Smart Nation (SmartTechCon)*, 1118–23.

Laplante, Phillip A. 2017. *Dictionary of Computer Science, Engineering, and Technology*. CRC Press.

Laplante, Phillip A, Mohamad Kassab, Nancy L Laplante, and Jeffrey M Voas. 2017. "Building Caring Healthcare Systems in the Internet of Things." *IEEE Systems Journal* 12 (3): 3030–37.

McCue, T J. 2015. "$117 Billion Market for Internet of Things in Healthcare by 2020." *Forbes Tech, April*.

Morgan, Steven. 2017. "Private Sector Audits and the Office of the Privacy Commissioner of Canada." *Int'l J. Data Protection Officer, Privacy Officer & Privacy Couns.* 1: 11.

Perrier, Elija. 2015. "Positive Disruption: Healthcare, Ageing and Participation in the Age of Technology."

Pointer, S C. 2014. "Australian Institute of Health and Welfare." *Canberra, Australia: Australian Institute of Health and Welfare.*

Shelby, Zach, and Carsten Bormann. 2011. *6LoWPAN: The Wireless Embedded Internet.* Vol. 43. John Wiley & Sons.

Soh, Harold, and Yiannis Demiris. 2015. "Learning Assistance by Demonstration: Smart Mobility with Shared Control and Paired Haptic Controllers." *Journal of Human-Robot Interaction* 4 (3): 76–100.

u Farooq, M, Muhammad Waseem, Sadia Mazhar, Anjum Khairi, and Talha Kamal. 2015. "A Review on Internet of Things (IoT)." *International Journal of Computer Applications* 113 (1): 1–7.

Ugrenovic, Dejana, and Gordana Gardasevic. 2015. "CoAP Protocol for Web-Based Monitoring in IoT Healthcare Applications." In *2015 23rd Telecommunications Forum Telfor (TELFOR)*, 79–82.

Ullah, Kaleem, Munam Ali Shah, and Sijing Zhang. 2016. "Effective Ways to Use the Internet of Things in the Field of Medical and Smart Health Care." In *2016 International Conference on Intelligent Systems Engineering (ICISE)*, 372–79.

Yadav, Lata, Sudhanshu Kumar, Anil KumarSagar, and Subrata Sahana. 2018. "Architecture, Applications, and Security for IOV: A Survey." In *2018 International Conference on Advances in Computing, Communication Control and Networking (ICACCCN)*, 383–90.

In: Intelligent Information Retrieval … ISBN: 978-1-68507-301-5
Editors: Parma Nand et al. © 2021 Nova Science Publishers, Inc.

Chapter 7

DATA PRIVACY AND SECURITY IN HEALTHCARE

Ruby Jain*, Ayush Kumar Singh and Sanskruti Rajore
Symbiosis Skills and Professional University, Pune, India

ABSTRACT

In recent years, the world has witnessed a data revolution. Each minute, terabytes of data is being generated. Whilst enjoying the perks of this data-driven society, a few challenges must also be addressed, i.e., storage, retrieval of data. Amongst which the major one has always been Data Privacy and Protection. Many organizations all around the world are dealing with similar concerns. A major part of which is the healthcare industry. They have been charged and prosecuted, numerously, for unauthorized data breaches leading to their pocket fill, using the patient's medical data (or medical history). Healthcare providers(workers/helpers) and their colleagues must protect the privacy of their patients and provide up to the mark services abiding by the regulatory specifications proposed by the Health Insurance Portability and Accountability Act of 1996 (HIPAA) [1] and additional norms, like the EU's General Data Protection Regulation (GDPR)[2]. Though these regulations may seem overwhelming, there are plenty of

* Corresponding Author's E-mail: ruby.jain81@gmail.com.

good practices and tools that a healthcare organization can use to ensure compliance. Advanced health security measures are aimed at adapting to emerging risks, addressing threats like privacy, security, and data protection during its movement, at rest, or in the process/s. This requires a multi-faceted, complex security proposition.

Keywords: Data, privacy, protection, medical, healthcare, security

INTRODUCTION

Driven by data i.e., patient records, compliance with regulatory requirements, and patient care, the healthcare industry is known for producing a large amount of data, over the years. This data has been stored in the form of hard copies. However, with digitization at its peak, the methods of storing data also revolutionized.

In the healthcare sector, big data is referred to as large and complex datasets, which are often difficult to manage. It is considered difficult to manage such data as it comprises a mixture of data types, the data comes in huge volumes and it continues to grow exponentially. The sum of information related to patient health and well-being constitutes "big data". Big data in the healthcare sector constitutes of clinical data from the CPOE and other platforms such as the decision support systems in the clinics (doctor's instructions, medical observations, laboratory data, pharmacy data, insurance policies, and other managing details); patient's data in the electronic patient records (EPRs); mechanical / sensor data, that is returned from monitoring critical signals; and little patient-related statistics, comprising of data from emergency cases, news headlines, and certain articles in medical journals.

Even though the expansion of big data usage in the healthcare domain has helped the medical sector evolve, there are still some loopholes in the system where big data fails. Year after year big data is questioned for its security and privacy due to the ever-growing count of healthcare methods, like clinical and offline communication, health data exchange, cloud computing, and so on. Healthcare organizations have discovered that a time-saving, cost-efficient, high-tech viewpoint to determine the safety and privacy protection requirements is not sufficient to protect the healthcare organization and its patients. To prevent the theft of sensitive patient information and several types of security breaches, effective, and efficient measures should be taken by all health organizations with due regard for future safety and privacy requirements. In this chapter, the threats to the protection of sensitive healthcare data and new technologies and solutions to these risks using new strategies will be discussed. We will focus on the issues of data security in healthcare, and list down several laws/regulations adopted by the various regulatory bodies all over the world and other appropriate methods and strategies that can be used to ensure patient privacy along with some case studies on healthcare data breaches.

DATA PRIVACY

Data privacy usually means a person's ability to decide for himself how much confidential information is to be shared with others, and to what extent. This personal information may be a person's name, location, contact details, or confidential information. Just as a person may wish to exclude someone from a private conversation, the majority of people intend to keep their records to themselves.

As the internet boosted over the years, so did the value of data. Websites, apps, and organizations often need to collect and store personal information about users to provide services. However, some organizations make sure to keep data security as their top priority. A few organizations may not provide adequate security around the data they collect, which may result in data breaches that endanger user privacy. Privacy is regarded as a fundamental human right, and data protection laws exist to protect that right. Data confidentiality becomes important for people to be willing to give in their data, they have to trust that their information will be handled with utmost caution. Organizations use several data protection techniques to gain the trust of their customers and users.

The past few years have witnessed the outbreak of constant threats and attacks on computer systems, with the chief goal of smuggling information. Numerous data breaches have occurred all through these with a steady upright angle. Every domain in the industry is facing this issue. The biggest data breach in history, with an approximation of over 200 million records being breached, was suffered by an American reporting agency in March of 2012. They had bought a firm named Court Ventures, that used public data to gather information. Court Ventures used to sell data to third parties on a regular basis. One of those third parties was a "Vietnamese fraudster service," that released the personal information of numerous Americans (which included their financial information and Social Security numbers) to its own customers [3]. Such examples can be found concerning every domain.

When data that must be kept confidential gets into the wrong hands, troublesome situations occur. Data breaches in a state-owned enterprise, for example, placing high-level confidential information in the hands of an enemy state. An infringement of the organization may place ownership data in the hands of a competitor. Breaking the law in a hospital or doctor's office can put patient health data in the hands of those who can abuse it [4]. Attacks on the privacy of patients are considered to be ever-growing distress in all the domains where an ocean of data is available, like healthcare where every second thousand and millions of records are being generated, thus making it challenging for the organization to keep a hold on it. Medical data breaches have real-world consequences. It's not about the 0's and 1's it's about people and lives.

As the number of data breaches increased, governments all around the world started putting strict regulations against such malpractices by placing strict laws like the General Data Protection Regulation established by the European Union.

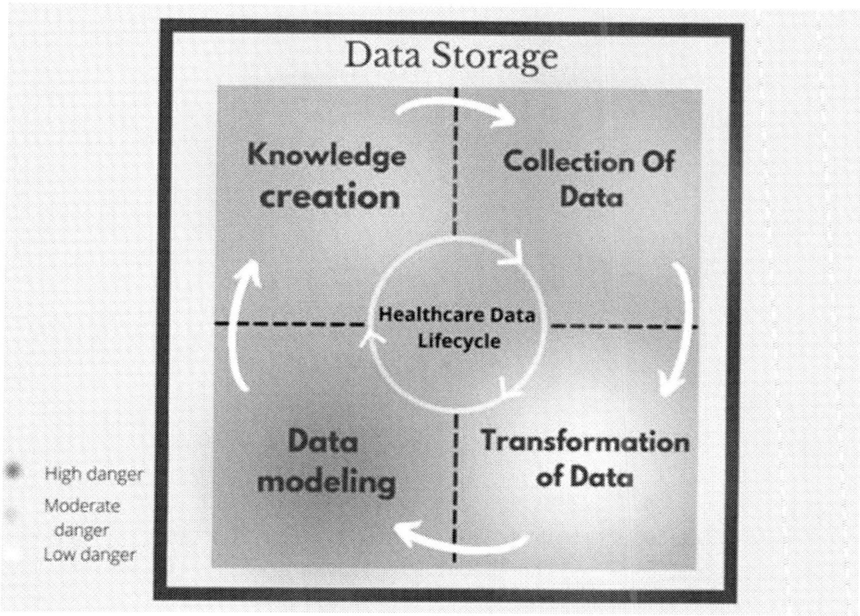

Figure 1. Risk Levels in data handling.

HEALTHCARE DATA BREACHES

A compilation of data breaches and the actual numbers were revealed, when the 'Health and Human Services Office for Civil Rights' started releasing statistics of medical data thefts on their website in 2009. In the section below charts are used to explain the trend of data breaches from October 2009 to 31st December 2020 [5].

Data Breaches by the Year

The chart below shows the relationship between incidents of data breaches with respect to every year, the trend clearly shows that ever since 2009 the count of data breaches each year has steadily increased

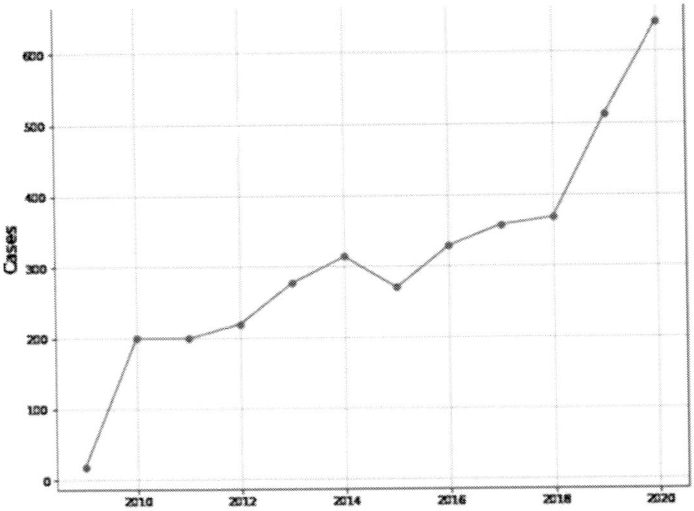

Note: These incidents include those data breaches where 500 or more records were exposed; These cases incorporate closed cases and the thefts that are still under investigation by the office of civil rights (OCR).

Figure 2. Records exposed by the Year.

Data Breaches: Based on Type of Breach

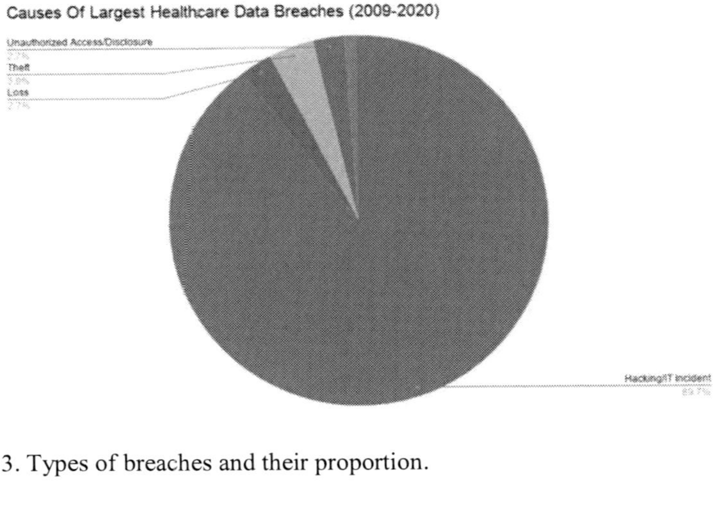

Figure 3. Types of breaches and their proportion.

It is evident that major causes of data breaches are:

1. Hacking/IT incident
2. Unauthorized access/disclosure
3. Theft

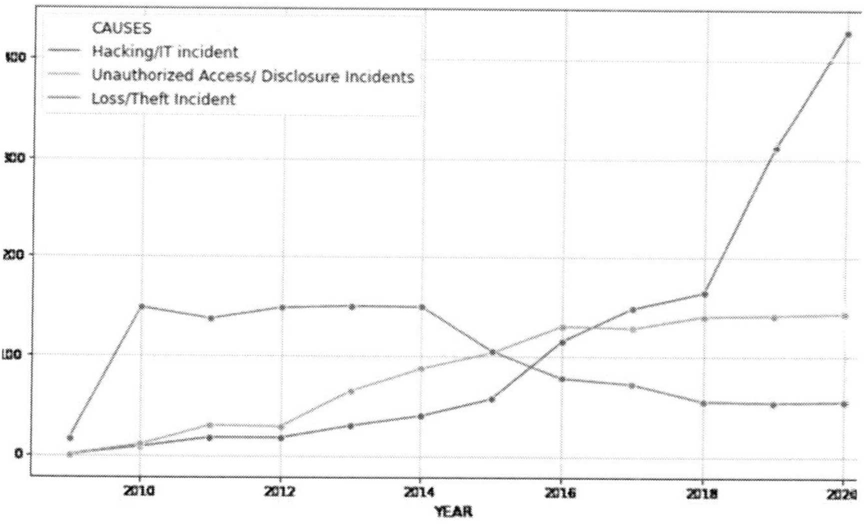

Figure 4. Comparative graph.

HACKING INCIDENTS

Hacking is one of the leading causes of data breaches in the medical sector, although it should be acknowledged that all sectors are getting better at detecting ransoms. Hacking/IT incidents were on the rise from 2014 to 2018 when most of the healthcare organizations failed to address these issues, some of these breaches went on for years before even being discovered.

UNAUTHORIZED ACCESS/DISCLOSURES

Just like IT incidents such as hacking, healthcare organizations are now quick to report any internal violations in the Office of Human Rights. These incidents contain human errors, negligence by the healthcare staff, or even disclosure by the will of the staff.

LOSS/THEFT OF PHI AND UNENCRYPTED EPHI

Integrated HIPAA organizations and business partners are now much better at securing patient data with managing controls that are both physical and technical such as encryption, although unlabeled electrical devices like laptops and mobile phones are unsafe in vehicles and public places. A vast majority of these cases of theft/loss include physical records such as documents or papers, which often lead to the disclosure of a lot of patients' healthcare data.

METHODS TO PROTECT HEALTHCARE DATA

Methods/measures that must be followed for the protection of healthcare data [6]:

Healthcare Staff Must Be Educated

The biggest threats to sensitive data in all domains remain human errors, but especially in this sector, a simple mistake or casual behavior can lead to major and costly repercussions for healthcare organizations. Awareness regarding data security can provide professionals with the necessary skills needed to make wise decisions and to exercise due diligence when dealing with such sensitive data.

Access to Database and Systems to Be Restricted

Introducing access controls can very well reinforce the safety of healthcare data by limiting access to it and specific applications for the users who only want to look into their services. System access restrictions require user's authentications, making sure that only permitted users can have entry into the sensitive information. Multiple levels of verifications are amongst some much-recommended techniques, it requires the users to substantiate that they are completely authorized to have access to certain sensitive information and systems using two or more than two authentication methods, such methods can be a password followed by a biometric scan.

Log, Monitor, and Control Usage

Data controls are beyond the scope of entry control and database monitoring to ensure that hostile data activity can be marked or obstructed in real-time. Healthcare organizations may use data controls to prevent certain actions involving sensitive data, such as web uploads, unauthorized email sending, copying to external drives, or printing. Data acquisition and classification play an important role in supporting this process by ensuring that sensitive information can be identified and tagged to achieve the appropriate level of protection.

Enabling providers and business partners to monitor which users access information, apps, and other resources, when, and from which devices and locations help maintain a record over data access. These logs appear to be important for audit purposes, helping organizations identify areas of concern and strengthening defenses when needed. In the event of an incident, the audit trail may allow organizations to identify accurate points of entry, determine the cause, and assess the damage.

Data to Be Encrypted

Encryption is one of the most effective ways to protect data from healthcare organizations. By encrypting information on the go and at rest, healthcare providers and business partners make it very difficult (impossible) for attackers to specify patient information or to access information.

Devices in Use to Be Secured

Healthcare providers and affiliated organizations use mobile devices while doing business, a doctor using a smart health device to gain knowledge that will assist them to manage patients having health insurance, or an admin services manager. Device security includes several security measures, including:

- Use of strong passwords.
- End-to-end encryption of data.
- Administrating mail accounts and file systems to prevent incidents of hacking or illegal data extraction.
- Guiding the users about the safety protocols to keep in mind at all times.
- Instructing the users to regularly update to the latest operating systems.
- Users should install antivirus software to keep them secure from dangerous malware.

Regular Risk Assessments to Be Conducted

Frequent risk evaluation may highlight risk or vulnerable areas in a healthcare company's safety, lack of staff education, inequalities in the safety of traders and the company's clients, and other subsequent reasons of concern. To better identify and minimize potential risks, periodically assessing the risk to the healthcare organization is a must, healthcare companies and their firm's partners can prevent menacing data breaches and several different kinds of harmful outcomes of data breaches, which may include damage to the reputation of the firm and large sums of penalties imposed by regulatory bodies.

Healthcare data is continuously being disseminated between contributors and affiliated organizations, making it easier to pay for and provide healthcare. Careful assessment of possible entrepreneurs becomes a really important safety regulation that healthcare companies must adopt.

To Backup Data to an Assured, Off-Track Place

Cyberattacks not only reveal crucial patient data but also jeopardize the integrity of the data. Even a natural mishap that affects a healthcare firm's data warehouse can have serious after-effects if the data is not stored and supported cautiously. This is why it is often recommended that data must be backed up, with strict encryption controls, authorization, and several safety measures to ensure its security. Offsite backups of the firm's data are essential for any sort of mishaps.

Laws for Data Protection in Several Countries

At the current times, it is critical that the medical sector supervise and take care of patient's personal information and address the underlying danger and licit obligations about the processing of personal information, also keeping in mind the growing complexity of effective data protection laws. Different nations have imposed several rules and policies regarding data protection, the rules and their key features for a few nations have been listed below in Table 1 [7].

Table 1. Laws for Data Protection

Nation	Rules	Noteworthy Features
United States of America	HIPAA Act Patient Safety and Quality Improvement Act	It needs the formation of governmental norms for the sale of electronic healthcare data. It provides the common man the right to confidentiality. Signed disclosure from stakeholders before handing any data about the provision of healthcare to anyone, including parents. People who violate privacy policies are held to public punishment. Safeguarding electronic health information.
European Union	Data Protection Directive	Protection of fundamental human rights, in particular the right to privacy of private information.
Canada	Personal Information Protection and Electronic Documents Act	Citizens are provided with the right to understand the reasons for the collection or usage of their data, thus organizations need to safeguard their information and use it honestly and cautiously.
United Kingdom	Data Protection Act	It gives citizens a method to limit their data. Private information can't be shared with a nation or region outside the European Economic Area until it guarantees an appropriate level of security of the rights of information.
Morocco	The 09-08 act.	Protection of data through the formation of a CNDP official by controlling the use of private and delicate information using data controls tools for any data refining operation.
Russia	Russian Federal Law on Personal Data	It needs data workers to follow all required directorial and technical actions to protect private information from unauthorized or coincidental access.
India	IT Act	Use of appropriate protection measures for sensitive data. It also provides reimbursement to people that suffered a loss. It assists for the arrest and/or fine to anyone who incurred improper loss or gains by revealing other's data while offering utility under the terms of a valid agreement.

Nation	Rules	Noteworthy Features
Brazil	Constitution	Intimacy, privacy, respect, and the status of the people are inescapable, and the guaranteed right to be brought in with physical or ethical damage caused by its non-obedience.
Angola	Data Protection Law	About the filtering of delicate information, managing and refining are permitted only where there is a legitimate law that allows such refining and prior authorization from the APD to be provided.

General Data Protection Regulation

GDPR was imposed by the EU Parliament in April 2016. GDPR aimed at replacing 'Data Protection Directive 95/46 / EC' in the spring of 2018 as the Supreme regulation, governing how firms safeguard the private data of EU citizens. The GDPR is a legalized substructure that imposes guidelines for the collection and processing of user data for people living in the European Union. As the law applies, no matter where websites are based, they have to abide by all the regulations mentioned in GDPR including the websites that attract European tourists or sell merchandise or services to European citizens. Some of the important requirements for General Data Protection Regulation includes:

1. Permission for data wrangling
2. Remove personal information like names to make the data anonymous
3. Notification about data breaches
4. Securely manage border data transfers
5. Certain firms have to hire a data protection officer who keeps a check to make sure all the regulations are being followed.

Under the GDPR's principles, when an organization collects personal data it has the full responsibility for the protection of the data from any sort of abuse or exploitation, if these organizations fail to protect it then they shall face large sums of penalties and lawsuits.

CASE STUDIES

Anthem Blue Cross

Since the rise of a data-driven world, there have been countless data breaches in the healthcare domain. Some of the biggest data breaches in the healthcare industry to date are stated. In February of 2015, Anthem, the largest healthcare firm in the United States of America, reported to the public and media that their computer systems have been hacked and the hackers had gained full access to their data warehouse and that 78 million personal identification information records including sensitive data like names, addresses, Dates of birth, medical IDs, and social security numbers were exposed to the hackers and were in peril to attacks. Investigators found out that Anthem employees were being assaulted by a cyber-army hacker's group associated with the People's Republic of China government; The groups "Deep Panda" and "Black Vine" had begun a large scale attack to blind-side consumers into fallacious sensitive mails which were linked to scam websites that compromised their services, by downloading malware which led to infecting their systems, and jeopardize many accounts all over the network until the hackers gained access to the firm's database comprising PII data. The firm spent around $230 million Just on eradicating the breach; which also included a cybersecurity insurance policy, fixing standard cases, and paying for additional security services and cyber protection.

Anthem also sent letters to 78.8 million customers that suffered by USPS and provided no charge credit monitoring services and ID protection services for 24 months. Anthem spent $115 million to resolve public action cases and bought an insurance policy from American International Group (AIG) worth $100 million to cover the collapse. It paid $ 2.5million to Mandiant to help with the inquiry and put forward a repair program. In addition to financial costs, Anthem also suffered serious vandalism to its businesses and their customers and was severely scrutinized by regulators [8].

The case of Anthem is a perfect example of how some loopholes in the system can cost a healthcare company big time. Lawsuits exceeding 100 filed against Anthem regarding this fraud were consolidated before Judge Koh. This was by far one of the biggest settlements of all time according to the lawyers working on the case [9].

Excellus Blue Cross

On September 9, 2015, Excellus Health Plan Inc. admitted to violating the data security rights of more than 10 million people. In October 2015, a case filed was against Excellus BlueCross BlueShield for failing to safeguard the patient records of Keller Rohrback L.L.P... On November 9, 2015, all linked cases awaiting in front of the United States District Court for the Western District of New York were compiled as a case called, 'Fero, et. al. v. Excellus Health Plan Inc., et al. (Rui Zhangand Ling Liu. 2010) [10].

The comprehensive combined complaint pursues allegations of class actions and the causes of the action under negligence, indifference, contract violations, breach of implied contract, improper enrichment, and certain Consumer Protection Laws in multiple states. The data breach led to certain settlements and penalties including a $5.1 million penalty for violation of confidentiality and protection laws mentioned in HIPAA. The Office for Civil Rights (OCR) declared that violated information included names, addresses, birth dates, email addresses, social security numbers, bank account details, health plan claims, and past medical details of all the patients. Punishment from the provincial jurisdiction comes as Excellus sustains to combat off the criminal act from those who suffered the happening. In which case, Excellus strived to proclaim that it was unfeasible for the information from the violation to be used for illegal intentions. Courts often reject that complainants in such cases should straight away connect the misuse of the data to the alleged violations.

The lawsuit, which is still pending in the U.S. District Court in the state of Western New York, stated that the ventures were incapable of preventing client data, took a lot of time to inform the clients regarding the violation, and failed to provide clients with appropriate details on how to safeguard themselves after the violation [11].

The Excellus penalty is amongst the largest costs paid to the OCR and it presents itself as a reminder to all the healthcare companies about their vulnerability to criminal hacking and data breaches.

CONCLUSION

According to a report by the International Data Corporation (IDC) sponsored by Seagate Technology, it is observed that big data is expected to expand faster in healthcare than in other fields such as manufacturing, financial services, or the media. The healthcare sector is growing at a rapid pace today due to the 2019 Coronavirus epidemic, and the need to manage patient care and information is also growing exponentially.

Thus data breaches are also increasing simultaneously, as shown in the records above. The threats due to hacking/IT incidents have increased in the past years, so it is essential to apply data protection schemes such as encryption and maintain data tracks.

Breaches due to theft, and unauthorized access/disclosure are also to be controlled and for this purpose, the stated methods of healthcare data protection must be practiced rigorously and with utter consciousness. Data is of utmost importance in today's world and it must be treated with care and caution while protecting its privacy.

It is readily apparent from the aforementioned points, the solitude and safety requirements for obedience with HIPAA depend not only on the services provided by the healthcare organization itself but also on any service providers conducting third-party business services. In other words, the consistency of a single organization depends largely on its capability to select and collaborate with firms involved in the same sturdy data prevention and safeguarding methods. In addition, healthcare organizations that prioritize data protection must understand that though HIPAA and other specified mechanisms are a fair initial point for the establishment of a data prevention system and avoiding high-cost punishments, efforts must go past compliance to ensure the safety of sensitive data from the modern menace.

REFERENCES

[1] Lane, Adrian. *Understanding and Selecting Data Masking Solutions: Creating Secure and Useful Data*, (Securosis Version 1.0, August 10, 2012).

[2] Hingwe, Kamlesh Kumar, S. Mary SairaBhanu, Sensitive Data Protection of DBaaS using OPE and FPE, 2014 (*Fourth International Conference of Emerging Applications of Information Technology,* 978-1-4799-4272-5/14 $31.00 © 2014 IEEE DOI 10.1109/EAIT.2014.22) Pg no. 320-327.

[3] Jain, Ruby Bhuvan, Dr. Manimala Puri, Umesh Jain. A Robust Dynamic Data Masking Transformation Approach to Safeguard Sensitive Data. February 2018, *International Journal on Future Revolution in Computer Science and Computer Engineering, volume: 4, issue: 2*. Pg no. 366-370.

[4] Abouelmehdia 1 Karim, Abderrahim BENI-HSSANEa, Hayat KHALOUFIa, Mostafa SAADIb. Big data security and privacy in healthcare: A Review, *the 8th International Conference on Emerging Ubiquitous Systems and Pervasive Networks (EUSPN 2017*)).

[5] Craig Terence & Mary E. Ludloff, *Privacy and Big Data.*

[6] *Indiana Health Information Exchange*: http://www.ihie.org/ (Accessed Date: March 24, 2016).

[7] Mcdonald, Carol, Transforming *Healthcare through Big Data, Strategies for leveraging big data in the healthcare industry.* Institute for health- 2013.

[8] Groves, Peter, Basel Kayyali, David Knott, Steve Van Kuiken, *The Big Data revolution in healthcare, accelerating value and innovation 2013.*

[9] CynergisTek, Redspin: *Breach Report 2016: Protected Health Information (PHI)* February 2017.

[10] Rui Zhangand Ling Liu:'' Security Models and Requirements for Healthcare Application Clouds'' (in *IEEE 3rd International Conference on Cloud Computing, 2010.*)

[11] Sweeney, L. "Achieving k-anonymity privacy protection using generalization and suppression," (in *the International journal on uncertainty, fuzziness, and knowledge-based systems,* vol. 10, 2002), pg. 571 – 588.

[12] Meiko Jensen, Challenges of privacy protection in Big Data Analytics 2013, (*IEEE International Congress on Big Data,* 2013).

[13] Xia, Xiaoling, Qiang Xiao and, Wei Ji (2012). An Efficient Method to Implement Data Private Protection for dynamic Numerical Sensitive Attributes, *The 7th International Conference on Computer Science & Education (ICCSE 2012) July 14-17, 2012.* Melbourne, Australia.

[14] Jain, Ruby, Dr. Manimala Puri, Securing Sensitive Business Data in Non-Production Environment Using Non-Zero Random Replacement Masking Method, *(International Journal of Application or Innovation in Engineering & Management (IJAIEM), Volume 8, Issue 3, March 2019*, ISSN 2319–4847), Pg no. 382-390.

[15] https://www.cdc.gov/phlp/publications/topic/hipaa.html#:~:text=The%20Health%20Insurance%20Portability%20and,the%20patient's%20consent%20or%20knowledge.

[16] https://digitalguardian.com/blog/what-gdpr-general-data-protection-regulation-understanding-and-complying-gdpr-data-protection.

[17] https://www.dataversity.net/brief-history-data-security/.

[18] https://www.analyticsinsight.net/data-privacy-important-comply-regulations/#:~:text=When%20customers%20give%20their%20personal,their%20employees%20from%20security%20breaches.
[19] https://www.hipaajournal.com/healthcare-data-breach-statistics/.
[20] https://digitalguardian.com/blog/healthcare-cybersecurity-tips-securing-private-health-data#:~:text=The%20HIPAA%20Privacy%20Rule%20%E2%80%93%20Requires,parties%20without%20prior%20patient%20authorization.
[21] https://www.sciencedirect.com/science/article/pii/S1877050917317015.
[22] https://www.nbcnews.com/news/us-news/anthem-pay-record-115m-settle-lawsuits-over-data-breach-n776246.
[23] https://medium.com/dataseries/take-out-how-anthem-was-breached-276b9ffca8da.
[24] https://krcomplexlit.com/currentcases/excellus-bluecross-blueshield-data-breach.
[25] https://www.cyberscoop.com/excellus-data-breach-fined-hhs-ocr/.
[26] https://digitalguardian.com/blog/top-10-biggest-healthcare-data-breaches-all-time.
[27] https://www.opswat.com/blog/11-largest-data-breaches-all-time-updated.

In: Intelligent Information Retrieval … ISBN: 978-1-68507-301-5
Editors: Parma Nand et al. © 2021 Nova Science Publishers, Inc.

Chapter 8

EXAMINING THE EFFECT OF ASHES OF VEDIC HOMA AND ITS SCIENTIFIC IMPACTS ON AQI WITH SOCIAL PERSPECTIVES: AN ML AND CPS BASED EXPERIMENTAL STUDY FOR DELHI-NCR ZONE AMIDST PANDEMIC THREATS

Rohit Rastogi[1,*], Sheelu Sagar[2,†], Neeti Tandon[3,‡] and T. Rajeshwari[4,§]

[1]Department of CSE, ABES Engineering College Ghaziabad, Ghaziabad, India
[2]Amity International Business School, Amity University, Noida, India
[3]Vikram University, Ujjain, India
[4]Yagyopathy Researcher and Active Social Volunteer, Kolkata, India

* Corresponding Author's E-mail: rohit.rastogi@abes.ac.in.
† Corresponding Author's E-mail: ssagar@amity.edu.
‡ Corresponding Author's E-mail: Tandon.neeti2019@gmail.com.
§ Corresponding Author's E-mail: simpleliving970@gmail.com.

Abstract

The present manuscript deals with the scientific analysis of Yajna and Mantra and it has been recorded that almost all the important chemical elements required for human health are present in Yajna ashes. Outdoor sensors have been used to measure the effect of Yajna process and it has been found that when the medicinal herbs and cow dung are used in Yagya, the ashes are more powerful and can be used for various purposes. Also it was observed that air quality was improved after the Yagya process. Critical Analysis and use of CPS based sensors like Outdoor Air Quality Monitor was used in the study.

Keywords: health care 4.0, AI, machine learning, sensor and IoT, Vedic science, Homa therapy, Yajna and Mantra, sensors

Introduction

Medicinal Plants

As per Atharva Veda, many medicinal plants are under use in Indian medical therapy. Param Pujya Guru Dev Pt. Sri Ram Sharma Acharya ji have told effect of Aayurved and importance of meditation on rising Sun. The infrared rays are more than 55% in the rising sun and that's health provider and protector (Pl. refer Figure 1 and Figure 2) (Zhilei Shan et al., 15 June 2020); (Chaturvedi, D. K. et al., 2013a).

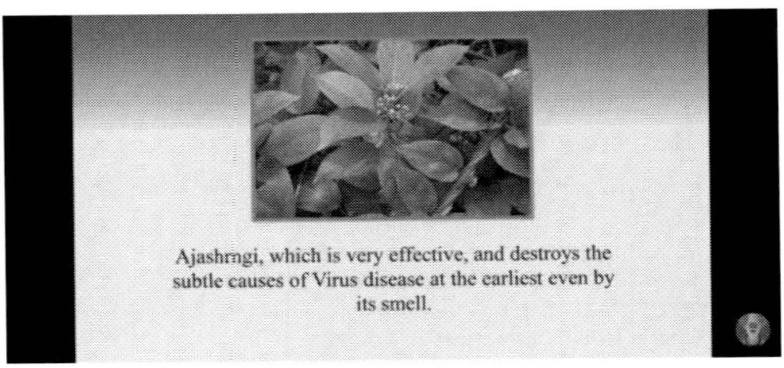
Ajashrngi, which is very effective, and destroys the
subtle causes of Virus disease at the earliest even by
its smell.

Figure 1. Ajashringi herbs, as elaborated in Aayurved.

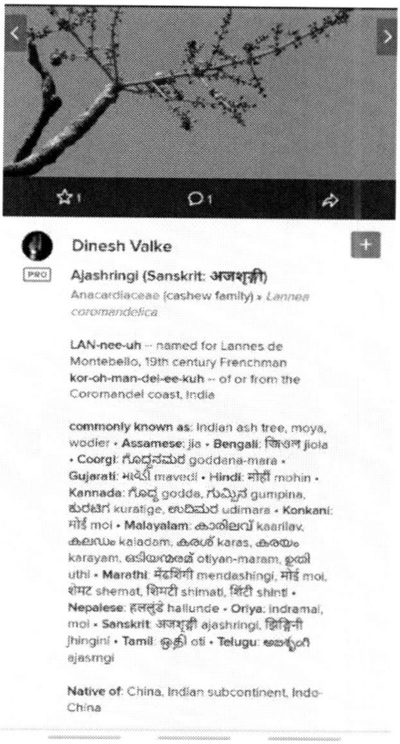

Figure 2. Botanical description of Ajashringi herbs, as elaborated in Aayurved.

The Sun Rays are the golden energizer; deadly destroys of virus and germs.

Yagya and Its Science

Cow Dung Based Kanda in Home and Its Ashes Purifies Water

Maximum content of oxygen in atmosphere is 21% but in any village of India, it is not more than 18 or 19% and in cities, it is merely around 11 or 12%. The fresh cow dung of Indian Breed cow, the life air oxygen content is 23%. When this cow dung is dried to make Kanda in sun then oxygen content is increased up to 27%. When this Kanda is burnt to make coal then Oxygen content is increased up to 30%. Again when this coal is converted to ashes after burning, then life-air is increased up to 46% (Cameron, A. J. et al., 2003); (Chaturvedi, D. K. et al., 2013b).

When this ash is burnt again to make super purified Ashes, then the life-air level reaches to 60%. Modern science says that if anything is processed many times, the mass and content is reduced. If this purified ash is dissolved 25 gm. Quantity in 10 lt. water then it helps to purify the water and all necessary elements are completed in that (Verma, S. et al., 2018); (Chaturvedi, D. K. et al., 2013c).

Agnihotra Ashes

If Agnihotra Gau (Cow) ashes are analyzed in lab then one will find it extremely useful for individual, family and society. Perhaps ancient Hindu Sages and saints offer these as Prasad to common people, visiting to them in their Ashram. One may also think when the extract of cow is so much useful then cow is also useful and that's why it has been termed as Gaumata in Indian Vedic scriptures and culture (Sharma, S. R., 2015a); (Gunavathi, C. et al., 2014) (Sharma, S. R., 2015a).

One should mix 10 to 15 gm. i.e., 3-4 tea spoon ash in one liter water, when this ash is settle down in bottom, then one can consume the water. It will remove all impurities of water and one will get many nutritious components. It is tested and verified by laboratory (Sharma, S. R., 2015b); (Kim, K. J. et al., 2019).

Element Form:

1. Oxygen O = 46.6%
2. Silicon SI = 30.12%
3. Calcium Ca = 7.71%
4. Magnesium Mg = 2.63%
5. Potassium K = 2.61%
6. Chlorine CL = 2.43%
7. Aluminum Al = 2.11%
8. Phosphorus P = 1.71%
9. Iron Fe = 1.46%
10. Sulphure S = 1.46%

11. Sodium Na = 1%
12. Titanium Ti = 0.19%
13. Manganese Mn = 0.13%
14. Barium Ba = 0.06%
15. Zinc Zn = 0.03%
16. Strontium Sr = 0.02%
17. Lead Pb = 0.02%
18. Copper Cu = 80 PPM
19. Vanadium V = 72 PPM
20. Bromine Br = 50 PPM
21. Zirconium Zr = 38 PPM

Oxide Forms:

1. Silicon Di Oxide -SIO2 = 64.44%
2. Calcium Oxide - CaO = 10.79%
3. Magnesium Oxide -MgO = 4-37%
4. Aluminum Oxide -AI2O3 = 3.99%
5. Phosphorus Penta Oxide -P2O5 = 3.93%
6. Potassium Oxide -K2O = 3.14%
7. Sulphur Oxide -SO3 = 2.79%
8. Chlorine CL = 2.43%
9. Iron Oxide -Fe2O3 = 2.09%
10. Sodium Oxide -Na2O = 1.35%
11. Titanium Oxide -TiO2 = 0.32%
12. Manganese Oxide -MnO = 0.17%
13. Barium Oxide -BaO = 0.07%
14. Zinc Oxide- ZnO = 0.03%
15. Strontium Oxide -SrO = 0.03%
16. Lead Oxide -PbO = 0.02%
17. Vanadium Oxide -V2O5 = 0.01%
18. Copper Oxide -CuO = 0.01%
19. Zirconium Oxide -ZrO2 = 52 PPM

20. Bromine Br = 50 PPM
21. Rubidium Oxide- Rb_2O = 32 PPM

To increase the Oxygen content in body, this cow dung ash is extremely useful.

SARS COVID-19

A document written by Chinese scientists and health officials before the pandemic in 2015 states that SARS corona viruses were a "new era of genetic weapons" that could be "artificially manipulated into an emerging human disease virus, then weaponries and unleashed, reported Weekend Australian (Sharma, S. R., 2015b); (Sharma, S. R., 2015a); (Mahajan, P., et al., 2016).

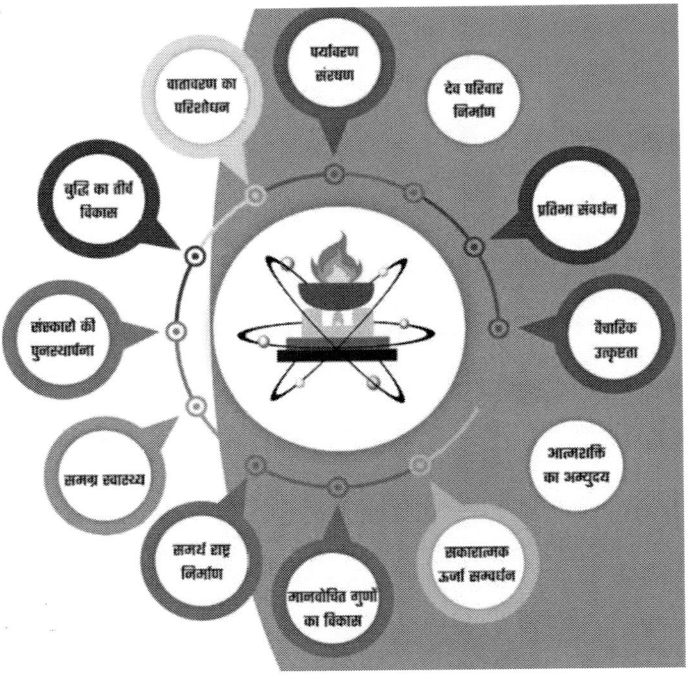

Figure 3. Positive Effect of Yajna in Various Dimensions.

These efforts are required to blame the right criminal. As another pandemic is on its way from China. And we are not been able to do anything. China has controlled this. Everyone as they have thermal imaging, face recognition software enabled security system. Here we don't even have oxygen or proper N-95 mask (Sharma, S. R., 2015a); (Marjani, M. et al., 2017).

Simple dhumra (Vapor) without Mantra is nothing the energy produced with a proper Vedic method is the true Yagya. So instead of trying salt or Neem to make situation worst do simple Yagya and Pranayama for minimum 10 minutes. Drink and apply Pranita Patra water and Ghee as its energy level become very high. Only the covered water should be used (Mistry, R. et al., 2020); (Sharma, S. R., 2015c).

As per scientists, a Diya has to be arranged and burnt below and above an oil diffuser, there we use stone salt, camphor that removes the negativity from the environment. But it is strictly restrained in Yajna. Neem Leaves (4 to 5) are sufficient. In Yagya, no salty things are allowed for oblations (Pl. refer Figure 3).

Mantra and Its Effects

Explanations for mantras, "you need pollution free, environment, full of positive energies, then first chant your first kalam from Quoran (ya ilahi villella, Mohammede rasullalla… what karma…). The meaning also says provoke my intellect into righteous path. Swaha is required for every oblations, (the way we feed our child, we say open your mouth "aaa.") with kalmar give 5 oblations first. Then 5 oblations on bhur, bhuvah swaha swaha. The 3 lokas, 1 where you stay and upper realms that will make you pollution free. This we are doing for sun, without him nothing is possible. Have faith and do. Same with Jains, their "naukara Mantra" with swaha, then on bhur bhuvaha swaha swaha (Sharma, S. R., 2015c); (Rastogi, R. et al., 2018a); (Sharma, S. R., 2015c).

There was one Jain retired professor from Bilaspur, Chattisgadh, India. He is Jain and tried Yagyopthy and his 35 year old illness he was expecting it to go away in 15 days. The team will also try to contact him see if he is still interested. All mantras got from Geet Sanjivani book, in a song (Saxena, M. et al., 2018) (as per Figure 3), (Gope, P. et al., 2016); (Rastogi, R. et al., 2018b).

LITERATURE SURVEY

In Aayurved texts (such as *Bhaishajya Ratnavali, Yog-ratnakar*), the inhalation of specific herbal medicinal-smoke *(Dhoomapana)* is recommended for therapeutic intervention for various conditions such as fever, pregnancy, poisonous animals' bites, etc. and for diseases such as mania, epilepsy, worm infections, syphilis, etc. The inhalation of medicinal-smoke of a specific herbal-powder combination of *neem* leaves (Melia azadirachta), *bach* (Acorus calamus), *kooth* (Saussurea lappa), *harad* (Terminalia chebula-Retz.), *saraso* (Brassica campestris-Linn.) and *googal* (Commiphora mukul-Engl.), destroys extreme fever in patients (Advait Danke, 2019).

In another example, the inhalation of the medicinal-smoke of a specific herbal-powder combination made using neem leaves, bach, hing (Ferula narthex-Boiss), sendha namak (Sodii chloridum), saraso was described to destroy worms, mange, and pus (Brahmvarchas, 1998); (Rastogi, R. et al., 2018c).

Yagya is a ritual like giving back to the atmosphere, whatever we have taken from it. Yagya also found an effective method to minimize the fungal load in a small area. Yagya smoke has potential to kill fungus like Aspergillus, Penicillium, Curvularia and Cladosporium, etc., grow in the polluted environment. These fungi cause fungal infection when mixed in the atmosphere (Rastogi, R. et al., 2019a).

Yagya helps to control pollution in the nearby area and kill and minimize these types of fungi. Thus, yagya is very beneficial to control the pollution and reduce the fungal infection and bacterial infection by reducing the fungi and bacteria present in the air by the help of yagya smoke generated by burning of samagri and substances (Gaurav Jain, 2017); (Gaurav Jain, 2019).

METHODOLOGIES AND EXPERIMENT SET UP

The instruments of high quality and accuracy have to be used in the experiment process. It was needed to measure the level of O2, CO2 etc. component density in a hall or campus before and after the Yagya activity.

Dr. Mamta Saxena used and found that PM and CO2 can be measured by Airveda device. It's good instrument and costs around INR 20000. The collected data for one month can be stored on cloud and can be downloaded anytime, its wifi compatible so one can see current data on one's mobile anytime.

It has 5 parameters PM2.5, PM 10, CO2, TEMP and HUMIDITY. (Rastogi, R. et al., 2019b)

Outdoor Sensors

Outdoor sensor devices are also available and they are costly and most of the time sensors are not reliable. The team used one such device on trial and used it for 2 months and compared with previous experiences. They found that one should use separate monitors for each gas like SO2, NO2, CO. They will work better. National Institute of Technology, Surat, Gujrat, India (Environment Section) and DSVV, Haridwar, India, they are using outdoor sensors to collect and record the data(Pl. refer Table 1) (Rastogi, R. et al., 2019c); (Rastogi, R. et al., 2020a).

Besides above sensor based info, the PureLogics lab India pvt. Ltd., Rohini, Delhi, India have developed a sensor and IoT based Device named as 'Portable Air Quality Monitor (Low Resolution).'

Table 1. Outdoor Sensor Specification

Gas Name	**Instr (RES) (PPB)**	**Range (PPB)**	**Sensor LOD**	**T90 Response**	**Reco'd Calibration**	**Expected Life**
Sensor Type	NDIR				Frequency	
Carbon Dioxide(CO2)	1 PPM	0-10,000 PPM	1 PPM	<20 S	12 months	5 Years
Sensor Type		Electrochemical				
Carbon Monoxide(CO)	1 PPB	0-1000 PPM	1 PPB	<30 S	12 months	3 Years
Ammonia(NH3)	1 PPB	0-100 PPM	1 PPB	<35 S	12 months	3 Years
Carbon disulfide (CS2)	<0.1 ppm	0-100 ppm	<0.1 ppm	<30 S	12 months	3 Years
Chlorine (Cl2)	20 PPB	0-20PPM	20 PPB	<60S	12 months	3 Years
Hydrogen chloride (HCl)	1 PPB	0-30 PPM	20 PPB	<70 S	12 months	3 Years
Sulfur dioxide (SO2)	1 PPB	0-100PPM	1 PPB	<60 S	12 months	3 Years
Nitric Oxide(NO)	1 PPB	0-20 PPM	1 PPB	<45 S	12 months	3 Years
Nitrogen dioxide (NO2)	1 PPB	0-20 PPM	1 PPB	<80 S	12 months	3 Years
Hydrogen Sulfide(H2S)	1 PPB	0-100PPM	1 PPB	<60 S	12 months	3 Years
Ozone(O3)	1 PPB	0-20 PPM	1 PPB	<80 S	12 months	2 Years
Oxygen(O2)	0.2%	0-25%	0.2%	<15 S	12 months	3 Years
Sensor Type	PID					
TVOC-Low PID	1 PPB	0-20 PPM	5 PPB	<5 S	12 months	5 Years
TVOC-High PID	0.1 PPM	0-10000 PPM	0.1 PPM	<5 S	12 months	5 Years

This device measures and produces data with attributes temperature, humidity, latitude, longitude, PM10, PM2.5, CO2, O3, NO2, SO2, CO and it's a lighter device with following specifications: weight of 420 Gm., Size 11X18X4 cm, Connectivity: GSM, Web Dashboard with remote data access, Mobile App Support: Android and IOS, Resolution of Particulate Matter: 1 micro gram/m^3, CO2-1PPM, NO2-1PPB, SO2-

1PPB, O3-1PPB, NO2-1 PPB, Warranty of Prodcut - 1 year on manufacturing defects, Device Calibration- 1 year after installation, Unit Cost 3,40,000 INR and GST and other taxes 61,200 INR so total price support: 401,200 INR.

Smart Air Quality Monitor

It is a multi dimensional device and important features are explained as follows.

Supports in Continuous Ambient Air Quality and Weather Monitoring

It incorporates multiple monitors into one space for comprehensive air quality, weather monitoring and pollution source locating (Pl. refer Figure 4).

Manages Your Air with Dashboard

With Prana air outdoor air quality monitor, one can access dashboard to view one's real time air quality readings and receive notifications.

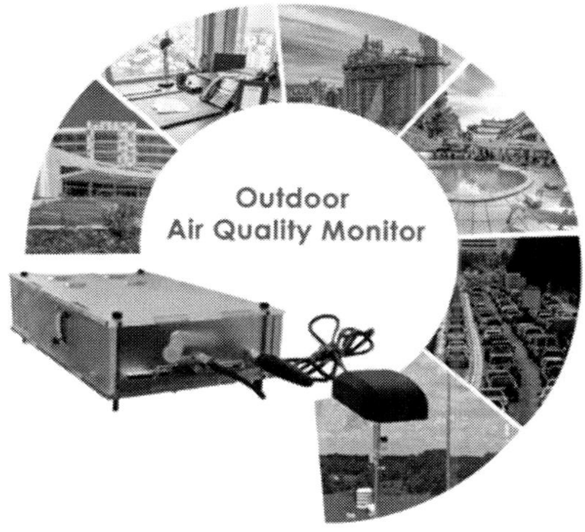

Figure 4. Outdoor Air Quality Monitor.

One can also use the dashboard with multiple devices, review and compare readings and export one's data to optimize one's space (Pl. refer Figure 5).

Sensor and Convenient Installation

Designed to fit into the standard junction box within the wall to enable quick and simple installation without complex engineering or construction (Pl. refer Figure 6, 7 and 8 for specifications).

RESULT ANALYSIS AND DISCUSSIONS

An Indoor Study was conducted in collaboration with central pollution Control Board, KG Marg, New Delhi, India, in the apartment of Dr. Mamta Saxena, a central Govt. officer and Yagyopathy researcher. Yajna was conducted in a room for about half an hour and air Microflora was sampled through gravity Settle method.

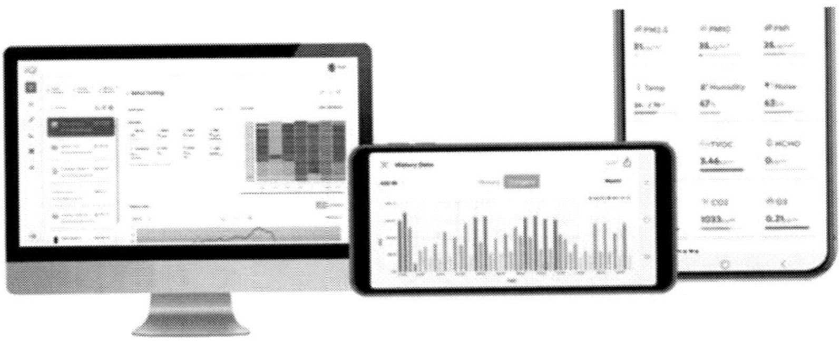

Figure 5. Dashboard display of outdoor air quality Sensor.

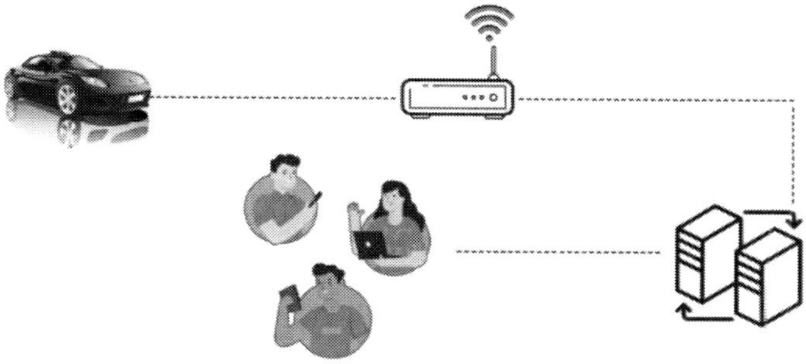

Figure 6. Flow chart of functioning of Out Door Air Quality Sensor.

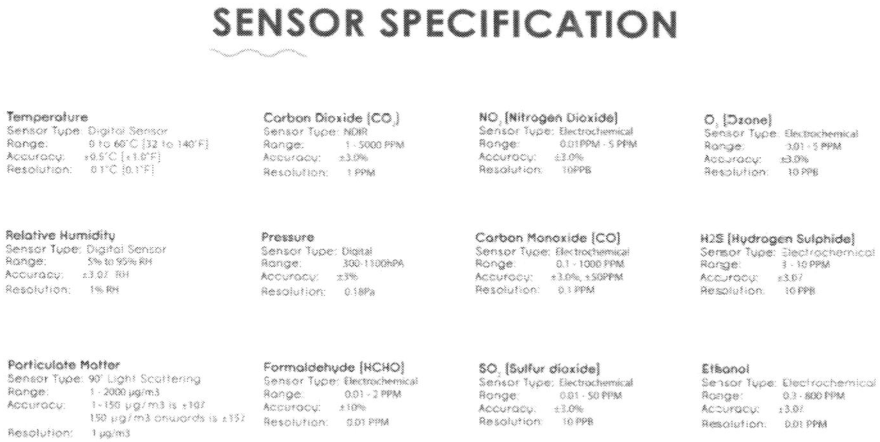

Figure 7. Sensor Specifications.

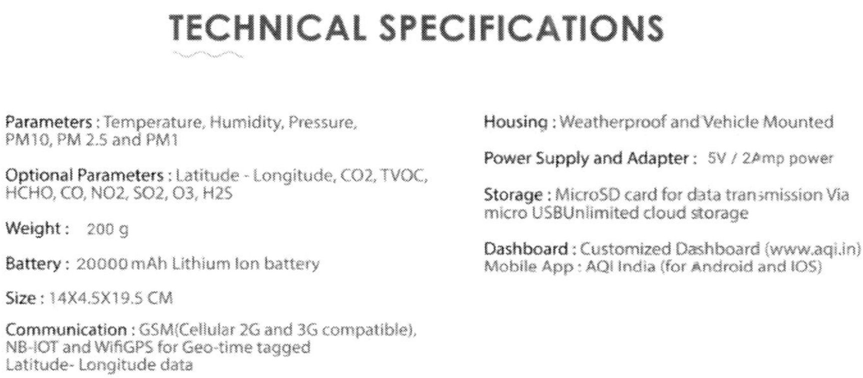
TECHNICAL SPECIFICATIONS
Parameters : Temperature, Humidity, Pressure, PM10, PM 2.5 and PM1
Optional Parameters : Latitude - Longitude, CO2, TVOC, HCHO, CO, NO2, SO2, O3, H2S
Weight : 200 g
Battery : 20000 mAh Lithium Ion battery
Size : 14X4.5X19.5 CM
Communication : GSM(Cellular 2G and 3G compatible), NB-IOT and WifiGPS for Geo-time tagged Latitude- Longitude data
Housing : Weatherproof and Vehicle Mounted
Power Supply and Adapter : 5V / 2Amp power
Storage : MicroSD card for data transmission Via micro USBUnlimited cloud storage
Dashboard : Customized Dashboard (www.aqi.in)
Mobile App : AQI India (for Android and IOS)

Figure 8. Technical Specifications.

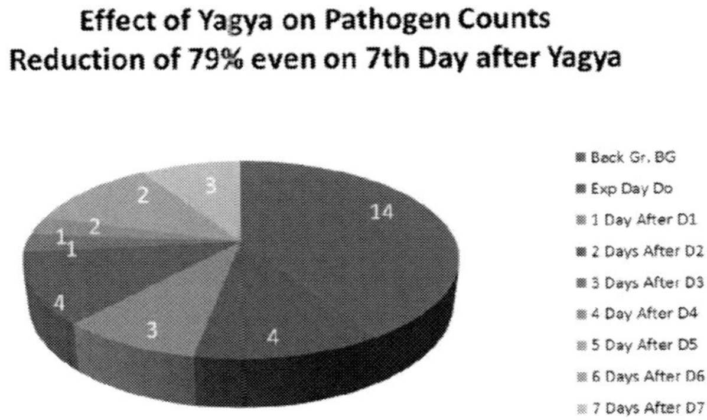

Figure 9. Effect of Yajna on Pathogens count Reduction of 79% even on the 7th Day of Yajna.

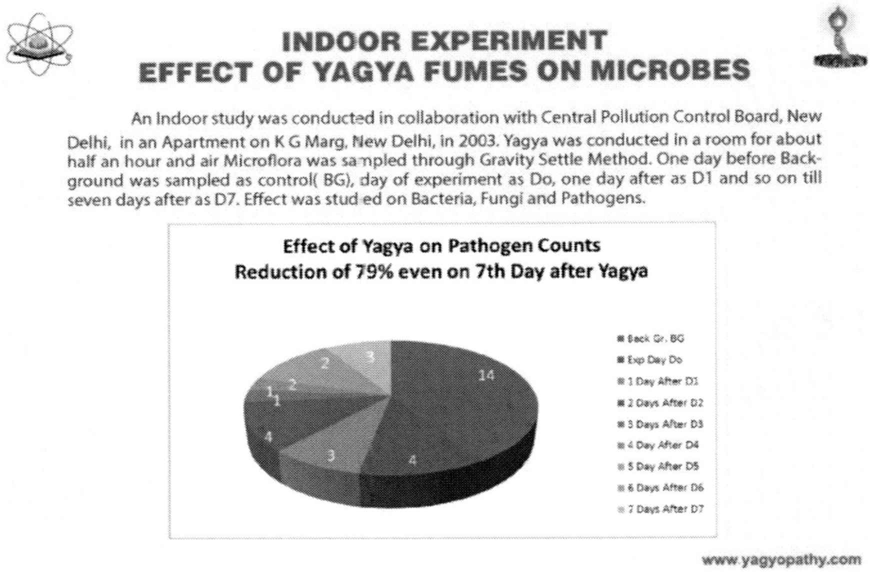

Figure 10. Indoor Study for Yagya vs. Non Yagya with Analysis of effect of Fumes on Bacteria.

One Day before background was sampled as controlled (BG), day of experiment as (DO), one day after as (D1) till after seven days, reading was done consecutively as (D7). Effect was studied on Bacteria, Fungi and Pathogens (Pl. refer Figure 9 and 10).

Indoor Study Results

Sr. Central Govt. officer in Min. of Statistics, New Delhi, India, Dr. Mamta Saxena Found in her experiments that after the Yajna activity, the content of Carbon mono Oxide, Carbon Di Oxide and pollutant Gases too. If Some Guggal, camphor and Havan Samagri is also used as oblation in slow fire, then some positive components are also emitted.

It has been also observed that some products are generated through Yagya activity compared to normal cleaning which make the atmosphere as bactereostatistic and it was found in research that the resonance is created in collective Yagya and this energy creates a mass and large effect in atmosphere. On 24, 25 and 26th May 2021, mass Yagya Activity was done in National Capital Region of India and its data was analyzed.

An active volunteer and researcher Ms. T. Rajeshwari also stated that Guggal, Desi camphor and clove should be mixed as a powder and use of it, smoke, mild fumigations are converted when you inhale you feel the expansion of your lungs. Mr. Anshul from Rudrapura, Uttarakhand and his team with joint collaboration with Cow Protection team and ABVP did a moving Yagya at the time of Pandemic so that its fume and vapors reach to every individual of that respective society (Pl. refer Figure 11).

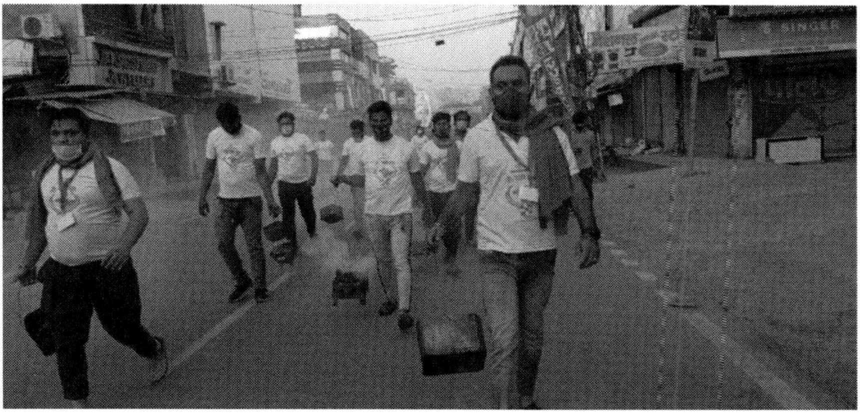

Figure 11. Moving Yagya at Rudrapur, Uttarakhand, India to purify environment during second wave of Covid'19 Pandemic.

Environment Purification through Yajna

Yajna is the basic foundation of Indian Culture and Rishi-Muni were organizing this Yajna ceremony to uplift common mass consciousness to heights. Havan process is cure therapy and atmosphere is filled with fragrance. It is best healing method for physical and mental illness.

Today, in pandemic and lockdown due to Sars-Cov'19, mass is bounded for online study and people are highly dependent on electronic gadgets. Havan is also helpful in curtailing the electromagnetic radiations emitting from these gadgets. It has been proved by scientists that 24 oblations of Gayatri Mantra and other few protocol based Mantra purifies our emotions and feelings, reduces the thought pollution.

The used cow-dung, mango woods, camphor, Agar, Guggal, Giloy, barley, Til etc. are made subtle in atmosphere and virus and bacteria are much diminished at significant level and it is maintained in atmosphere for sufficient time. Poisonous gases like O2, CO, SO2, NO2 are heavily improvised and reduced. Today many scientific experiments are going on this process. Dev Sanskriti University of Shantikunj Haridwar, India is outstanding institute on the researches based on Homa Therapy (Pl. refer Figure 12 and Figure 13).

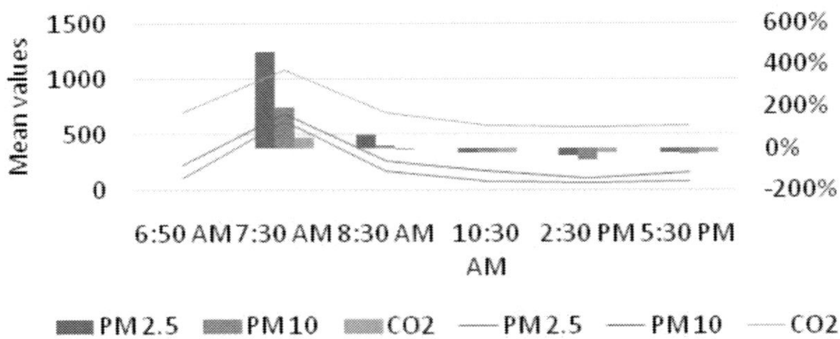

Figure 12. Comparative Emission Reduction Capacity (Mango Wood vs. Gomay Samidha) - Part 1.

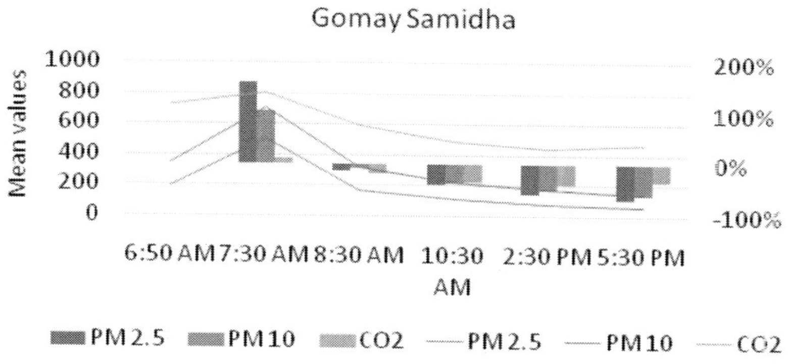

Figure 13. Comparative Emission Reduction Capacity (Mango Wood vs. Gomay Samidha) - Part 2.

- To check the PM effect and gaseous pollution inside the home, following experiments were done.
- Effect of Yajna by Gomay (cow-dung) based Samidha inside room.
- Effect of Yajna by mango wood based Samidha inside room and effect on PM2.5, PM10, CO, CO2 with help of Airveda device.
- Effect of emitted CO2 and effect of Kalash water.
- Total experiments on mango wood were four and total experiment on Gomay Samidha was Four.

Analysis of Results

The derivations from all the experiments were as below:

- Control on Pollution by Cow-dung based Samidha over mango wood was comparatively higher especially on PM2.5 and PM10.
- Cow dung Samidha was used with quantity 30 gm. To conduct whole Yajna activity but the mango wood quantity should be 130 to 150 grams.
- Clove of cow was used up to 20-30 grams and around 30-40 gm. Havan samagri of herbs was used.

- The amount of CO and other pollutant gaseous elements was at minimum level before taking Yajak (person doing Yajna) one's position.
- It was found to keep the water vessel (Kalash) at heights of 2 feet in Yagyashala that the level of CO2 was continuously decreasing.

RECOMMENDATIONS

I am wondering; do we really need to prove benefits of Yagya and show results in equipment, I don't think so. The time has come when people will realize and adopt this wisdom created in Vedic Sanskriti. Why to prove? It is their ignorance who wants to see the results and those ignorant will always be like that. Time will teach them. Just a thought. But wise thinking says that there are many myths also being circulated in respect of Havan.

Once we have experimented and tested they can be dispelled and also one comes to know the right way of doing Yagya. One myth which I have been hearing is that tons of oxygen is produced during yagya done with Cows clove. But this is not correct. The team has checked with oxygen device and it is incorrect. So, there are audiences who just say what they want. They need to get it clear. The manuscript helps to provide them a scientific way of thinking with actual facts (Rastogi, R. et al., 2020b).

NOVELTY OF WORK

Though the Hindu Vedic literature is highly scientific yet less efforts have been done to prove its validity and authentication. Through manuscript the scientific aspect and benefits have been highlighted. The ashes of different woods and cow dung are being lab tested and their results are displayed and humanity can get its benefits (Saxena, M. et al., 2020).

Future Research Directions and Limitations

Many researches are going on for rain cloud inviting through Yagya, Agriculture improvement and mental and physical fitness. One may contribute on these aspects of this dimension of this Vedic science. It has been also found that Yagya process also cleans the environment and no. of bacteria and pathogens have been drastically controlled and even after seven days of activity the positivity through negative ions were maintained (Rastogi, R. et al., 2020c); (Saxena, M. et al., 2008).

Conclusion

The manuscript detailed discussed about the critical analysis of Yagya ashes and Mantra effects. High level of mental and physical fitness has been also observed through this therapy. In whole world, it is being treated as Yagyopathy. The humanity and whole scientific fraternity is now fascinated towards its glorious benefits and science is widely accepting it. The manuscript contains the benefits of Yajna Ashes in different dimensions. Now days, the Yagya Activity has been considered as the prominent therapy for many disease control.

References

[1] Cameron, A. J., Paul Z Zimmet, David W Dunstan, Marita Dalton, Jonathan E Shaw, Timothy A Welborn, Neville Owen, Jo Salmon, Damien Jolly, (5 May, 2003); *Overweight and obesity in Australia: the 1999-2000 Australian Diabetes, Obesity and Lifestyle Study (AusDiab)*; https://doi.org/10.5694/j.1326-5377.2003.tb05283.x.

[2] Verma, S. Mishra, A., Shrivastava, V. (2018). Yagya Therapy in Vedic and Ayurvedic Literature: A Preliminary exploration, *Interdisciplinary Journal of Yagya Research*, 1(1), pp. 15-20. http://ijyr.dsvv.ac.in/index.php/ijyr/article/view/7/13.

[3] Shan, Zh., Yanping Li, Megu Y. Baden; *Association between Healthy Eating Patterns and Risk of Cardiovascular Disease*; June 15, 2020; https://jamanetwork.com/journals/jamainternalmedicine/article-abstract/2767106.

[4] Sharma, S. R. (2015a). *Shabd Brahma-Naad Brahm,* Page - 4, 27, 62, 63, 69, 81, 119.

[5] Sharma, S. R. (2015b). *Gayatri MahaVigyan,* Page - 4.

[6] Sharma, S. R. (2015c), *Pandit Shree Ram Sharma ji Aachary Vangmay* - 26, Yagya, ek Samagra Upchar, Page 4.2, 4.26.

[7] Danke, A. (Oct., 23, 2019). Blog- Scientific & Ayurvedic perspective of Yagya/Hawan & it's benefits, *BodhMarga Foundation*, Wellness Vibe URL- https://medium.com/@advaitdanke/scientific-ayurvedic-perspective-of-yagya-havan-its-benefits-8ef621999ed8.

[8] Brahmavarchas, (1998). Editor. Hindu Dharm mein yagyon ka sthan tatha prayojan (Hindi). In: *Yagya ka gyan-vigyan* (Pt Shriram Sharma Achraya Vangmay No 25). Akhand Jyoti Sansthan, Mathura-281003; pp. 2.67-2.71.

[9] Jain, G., (2017). *Blog - Hawan for Cleansing the Environment* URL- https://medium.com/@giftofforest192/hawan-for-cleansing-the-environment-a9e1746e38e0.

[10] Jain, G., (5 Sept. 2019). *Yagya Ayurveda,* URL-https://www.facebook.com/yagyaayurved/.

[11] Gope, P., Tzonelih Hwang (2016). *BSN-Care: A Secure IoT-Based Modern Healthcare System Using Body Sensor Network*; March 1, 2016; http://dl.papergram.ir/mobileapp1/iot/202/h209.pdf.

[12] Chaturvedi, D. K., and Arya, M. (2013a). A Study of Correlation between Consciousness Level and Performance of Worker, *Industrial Engineering Journal* 6 (8), pp. 40-43.

[13] Chaturvedi, D. K., and Arya, M. (2013b). Correlation between Human Performance and Consciousness, *IEEE-International Conference on Human Computer Interaction,* 23-24 Aug. 2013, Saveetha School of Engineering, Saveetha University, Thandalam, Chennai, IN, India.

[14] Chaturvedi, D. K., and Satsangi, R. (16 Nov. 2013c). The Correlation between Student Performance and Consciousness Level, *International Conference on Advanced Computing and Communication Technologies (ICACCT™-2013),* Asia Pacific Institute of Information Technology SD India, Panipat (Haryana), Souvenir – pp. 66, proc. pp. 200-203.

[15] Gunavathi, C., and Premalatha, K. (2014). A Comparative Analysis of Swarm Intelligence Techniques for Feature Selection in Cancer Classification, *The Scientific World Journal,* 14, Pages: 12.

[16] Kim, K. J., and Tagkopoulos, L. (2019). Application of Machine Learning Rheumatic Disease Research, *Korean J. Intern Med.,* 34, page no.:2.

[17] Mahajan, P. (May 2016). Application of Pattern Recognition Algorithm in Health and Medicine: a review, *International Journal of Engineering and Computer Science,* 5(5), page no: 16580-83.

[18] Marjani, M., Nasaruddin, F., Gani, A., Karim, A., Hashem, I. A. T., Siddiqa, A., and Yakoob, I. (March 2017). Big IoT Data Analytics: Architecture, Opportunities, and Open Research Challenges, *IEEE Access*, 5, Page: 5247-5261.

[19] Mistry, R., Tanwar, S., Tyagi, S., and Kumar, N. (2020) Blockchain for 5G-Enabled IoT for Industrial Automation: A Systematic Review, Solutions, and Challenges, *Mechanical Systems and Signal Processing*, 135, pp. 1-19.

[20] Rastogi, R., Chaturvedi, D. K., Sharma, S., Bansal, A., and Agrawal, A. (14th-16 March, 2018a). Audio Visual EMG & GSR Biofeedback Analysis for Effect of Spiritual Techniques on Human Behaviour and Psychic Challenges, in *Proceedings of the 12th INDIACom; INDIACom-2018;* pp 252-258.

[21] Rastogi, R., Chaturvedi, D. K., Satya, S., Arora, N., Sirohi, H., Singh, M., Verma, P., and Singh, V. (14-15 December 2018b). Which One is Best: Electromyography Biofeedback Efficacy Analysis on Audio, Visual and Audio-Visual Modes for Chronic TTH on Different Characteristics, in *the proceedings of International Conference on Computational Intelligence & IoT (ICCIIoT) 2018*, at National Institute of Technology Agartala, Tripura, India, ELSEVIER-SSRN Digital Library (ISSN 1556-5068).

[22] Rastogi, R., Chaturvedi, D. K., Satya, S., Arora, N., Saini, H., Verma, H., and Mehlyan, K. (14-15 December 2018c). Comparative Efficacy Analysis of Electromyography and Galvanic Skin Resistance Biofeedback on Audio Mode for Chronic TTH on Various Indicators, in *the proceedings of International Conference on Computational Intelligence & IoT (ICCIIoT) 2018,* at National Institute of Technology Agartala, Tripura, India, ELSEVIER-SSRN Digital Library (ISSN 1556-5068).

[23] Rastogi, R., Saxena, M., Sharma, S. K., Muralidharan, S., Beriwal, V. K., Singhal, P., Rastogi, M., and Shrivastava, R. (13-14 Dec. 2019a). Evaluation of Efficacy of Yagya Therapy on T2- Diabetes Mellitus Patients, in *the proceedings of The 2nd edition of International Conference on Industry Interactive Innovations in Science, Engineering and Technology (I3SET2K19)* organized by JIS College of Engineering, Kalyani, West Bengal, https://papers.ssrn.com/sol3/papers.cfm?abstract_id=3514326.

[24] Rastogi, R., Saxena, M., Gupta, U. S., Sharma, S., Chaturvedi, D. K., Singhal, P., Gupta, M., Garg, P., Gupta, M., and Maheshwari, M. (13-14 Dec. 2019b). Yajna and Mantra Therapy Applications on Diabetic Subjects: Computational Intelligence Based Experimental Approach, in *the proceedings of The 2nd edition of International Conference on Industry Interactive Innovations in Science, Engineering and Technology (I3SET2K19)* organized by JIS College of Engineering, Kalyani, West Bengal, https://papers.ssrn.com/sol3/papers.cfm?abstract_id=3515800.

[25] Rastogi, R., Saxena, M., Sharma, S. K., Murlidharan, S., Berival, V. K., Jaiswal, D., Sharma, A., & Mishra, A. (13-14 Dec. 2019c). Statistical Analysis on Efficacy of Yagya Therapy for Type-2 Diabetic Mellitus Patients through Various Parameters. In: Das A., Nayak J., Naik B., Dutta S., Pelusi D. (eds) *on Computational Intelligence in Pattern Recognition (CIPR), Kalyani, West Bengal. Advs in Intelligent Syst., Computing,* Vol. 1120, Computational Intelligence in Pattern, Recognition, 978-981-15-2448-6, 487895_1_En, (15), doi: https://10.1007/978-981-15-2449-3_15, 181-197.

[26] Rastogi, R., Chaturvedi, D. K., Verma, H., Mishra, Y., & Gupta, M. (2020a). Identifying Better? Analytical Trends to Check Subjects' Medications Using Biofeedback Therapies, *IGL Global, International Journal of Applied Research on Public Health Management (IJARPHM:* 5(1), Article 2. doi: https://10.4018/IJARPHM.2020010102, pp. 14-31, ISSN: 2639-7692|EISSN: 2639-7706|doi: https://10.4018/IJARPHM, https://www.igi-global.com/article/identifying-better/240753.

[27] Rastogi, R., Gupta, M., & Chaturvedi, D. K. (2020b). Efficacy of Study for Correlation of TTH vs Age and Gender Factors using EMG Biofeedback Technique, *International Journal of Applied Research on Public Health Management (IJARPHM)* 5(1), Article 4., pp. 49-66, doi: https://10.4018/IJARPHM.2020010104.

[28] Rastogi, R., Chaturvedi, D. K., Satya, S., Arora, N., Gupta, M., Verma, H., & Saini, H. (2020c). An Optimized Biofeedback EMG and GSR Biofeedback Therapy for Chronic TTH on SF-36 Scores of Different MMBD Modes on Various Medical Symptoms, *in Studies Comp. Intelligence,* Vol. 841,: Hybrid Machine Intelligence for Medical Image Analysis, 978-981-13-8929-0, 468690_1_En, (8) (2020c). S. Bhattacharya et al., (eds.), https://doi.org/10.1007/978-981-13-8930-6_8.

[29] Saxena, M., Sengupta, B., & Pandya, P. (Sept. 2008). Controlling the Microflora in Outdoor Environment: Effect of Yagya, *Indian Journal of Air Pollution Control,* 8(2), pp. 30-36.

[30] Saxena, M., Kumar, B., & Matharu, S. (Oct. 2018). Impact of Yagya on Particulate Matters, *Interdisciplinary Journal of Yagya Research,* 1(1), pp. 01-08.

[31] Saxena, M., Sharma, S. K., Muralidharan, S., Beriwal, V., Rastogi, R., Singhal, P., Sharma, V., & Sangam, U. (4th-5th January, 2020). Statistical Analysis of Efficacy of Yagya Therapy on Type-2 Diabetic Mellitus Patients on Various Parameters, In *Proceedings of 2nd International Conference on Computational Intelligence in Pattern Recognition (CIPR – 2020),* Institute of Engineering and Management, Kolkata, West Bengal, India.

In: Intelligent Information Retrieval … ISBN: 978-1-68507-301-5
Editors: Parma Nand et al. © 2021 Nova Science Publishers, Inc.

Chapter 9

NLP: SMART TEXTING SYSTEM BASED ON ANDROID

Frankly Chauhan, Jatin Kumar, Chandan Sahu, Subrata Sahana* and Anil Kumar Sagar
Department of Computer Science and Engineering,
Sharda University, Greater Noida, India

ABSTRACT

Designing a device like a human which shows human behavior, particularly the capacity of speaking and responding naturally, increase the interest of engineers and scientist. Since the 1930s, the problem of speech and text recognition has been approached progressively because a bell lab scientist HOMER-DUDLEY proposed a system model for speech recognition. For natural language, we need to convert a simple device or machine into a well-sophisticated machine so that a speech can effectively produce. In this, we mainly focus on major points in the development of automatic speech and text recognition. Our text conversion is also a factor used in speech recognition for the last few years.

Technique to process improved text-to-speech is disclosed, this improved technology converts the electronic document of our text into

* Corresponding Author's E-mail: subrata.sahana@gmail.com.

audio output which includes both speeches associated with our text as well as from our audio clip. Applying NLP-based data extraction techniques can automatically help the users. Cues to the listener when m/c produced output in a speech about a document. Before a text-to-speech conversion, our audio contextual cue is based on a document. The audio file of a document can be given to the user so that the user can hear all the documents rather than reading text.

Keywords: Natural Language Processing (NLP), Speech to Text, Text to Speech, Query Support System, Document Conversion, Unstructured Data

INTRODUCTION

We know that mobile phones are an indispensable source of communication used in modern society for the past few years. We can send text messages and can make a call from a place to another, easily. Phone calls fulfill a gap over long-distance communication easily. (Trivedi et al. 2018) A path-breaking innovation has been recently seen, where voice messages are being converted into voice messages. In this chapter, we are going to see different types of Natural Language Processing applications like a Query support system, unstructured data, Document and data conversion, and text to speech and speech to text conversion (Prasad 2015).

Android Devices

Now a day we are using different kinds of virtual personal assistants (like SERI, CORTANA, and GOOGLE) on our Android devices. (Bandhu, Singh, and Sanjay 2019) And these mentioned devices are evolving at a very fast pace with the performance of a system, their efficiency, and the working of these machines. But as we know that all such personal assistant uses internet connectivity for their access. They have a huge size of datasets to communicate and to store data that cannot be stored offline, so we need online storage like cloud services. We very much depend on Internet but it is also costly, so we have decided that we develop software and hardware so that users can access her voice command without using the Internet (Trivedi et al. 2018).

Text to Speech Recognition

In the given flow chart, we show how to convert text to speech in which we show that firstly we should analyze the data then process it, understood, and then our text is converted into audio (Bandhu, Singh, and Sanjay 2019).

The system works in 5phases as shown in Figure 1:

- Speech Input
- Speech Processing
- Feature Extraction
- Task Execution
- Text to Speech.

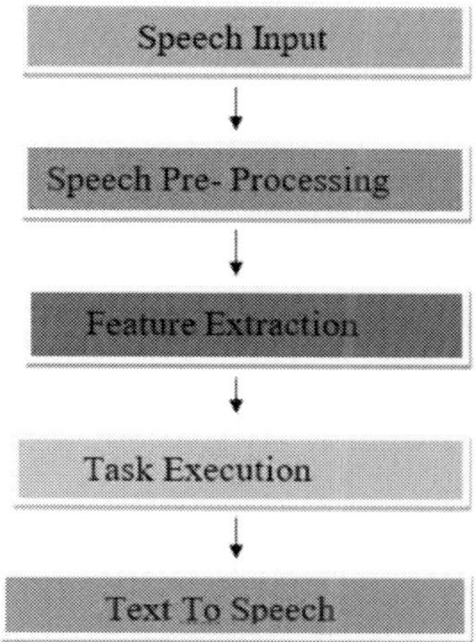

Figure 1. Flow diagram of offline android smartphones (Bandhu, Singh, and Sanjay 2019).

Speech to Text Recognition

Voice is the most common way of communication process for people to pass the message to each other. Now day's voice processing technologies are an interesting task but are limited also. Because of this processing, devices are responding correctly to human voice and provide an interface to use the valuable services of machines. "Speech-to-text," allows the machine to translate human voice requests and dictation into text form. Speech recognition system: - speech-to-text is a process in which speech converting an acoustic signal which is captured using a microphone into a set of words. (Trivedi et al. 2018) These recorded data are going to be used for document preparation. Human speech is a common method of communication in our societies. (Ifeanyi, Ikenna, and Izunna 2014) To convert Speech-to-text input taken from the microphone in the form of speech and then it is converted into the text from which is displayed on the desktop. In speech recognition technology, we process our voice and also study our voice signals (Khilari and Bhope 2015).

BRIEF HISTORY

We all are much familiar with the famous speech recognition research. Two very famous application is used in these days i.e., Google Assistant and Apple's SIRI. These are all new advents though brought about by rapid advancement in technology (Bakiri 1991).

Our exploitation of speech recognition goes way back to the 1950s. So, our speech recognition technique develops over 50 years ago. We prepare a neat and clean timeline chart for you to show how speech and text recognition systems have evolved over the years as described in Figure 2.

- In 1952: In 1952, the first speech recognition system Audrey was developed by three Bell Labs researchers named Audrey. In those days Audrey was designed to recognize only digits.

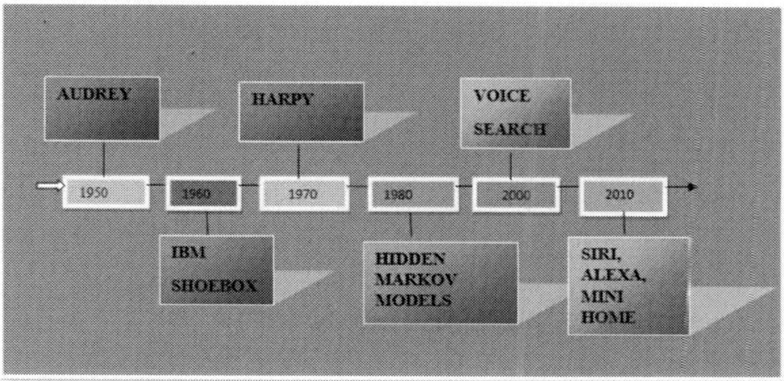

Figure 2. History of development in NLP: Text to Speech and vice versa (Mahanta et al. 2016; Shih and Sproat 1996).

- IN 1966: Linear predictive coding, 1966 began development with the work of Fumitada Itakuru of University of Nagoya and Shuzo Saito of Nippon telegram, telephone (NTT) in 1966.
- 1970-1990: Within 10 years our IBM came up with her first speech recognition system- "IBM Shoebox," which can recognize 16 words including digits. You can add the values by this also, like to add 6, 8, 5 you got your correct answer.
- 1971: Our DARPA agency which is called "The Defense Advanced Research Projects Agency" contribute a lot to speech recognition technique development and also gave funds to a program named "Speech Understanding Research" for 5 years from 1971. And one popular achievement is also there which is called "Harpy" at that time.
- 1972: A conference in Newton, Massachusetts which is conducted by IEEE Acoustics which is a speech and signal, processing group.
- 1976: ICASSP has been a major venue for the publication of the speech recognition system which was held in Philadelphia in 1976.
- 1982: Dragon systems was one of IBM's few competitors
- 1987: In 19287, recognizer from Kurzweil Applied Intelligence.

Table 1. Descriptive Survey on Text to speech recognition and vice versa

Author(s) Name	Year	Chapter name	Technique	Results
Kuldip K. Paliwal	2004	Use of Dynamic spectral for the recognition of Noisy speech.	In this report, they use Spectral Sub-band Centroids.	They show the feature of the SSC coefficient which is more resilient to noise than the MFCC features.
Esfandiari Zavareheri	2005	Restoration of short-time DFT trajectories using Kalman filters for Speech Enhancement.	They use two semantic-lexical and joint semantic lexical modeling with concept sequence modeling.	Tightness of integration between lexical and semantic items and also increase the level of semantic information utilized.
Ibrahim Patel	2010	Use of MFCC for spectral Decomposition technique and use HMM for speech recognition.	Resolution Decomposition with separating frequency is the mapping approach.	It shows the learning accuracy for speech recognition and how you improve quality metrics of speech recognition using computational time.
Kavita Sharma	2012	Speech Denoising using various types of Filters.	Wavelets, Filters, IIR, FIR, and so on.	We want clear speech and noise for speech enhancement so we use filters in speech recognition.
Shanker Dev Dhingra	2013	Use of MFCC and DTW for Isolated speech Recognition.	DTW (Dynamic Time Warping.	For speech identification, fast computing speed, and minimum error rates can be done by DTW which is the best non-linear feature matching technique.

- 1990: A consumer product released in 1990 known as Dragon Dictate. In 1990, telephone calls without the use of human being service are developed by AT&T.
- In 2001: A user can search queries by speaking to your machine because Google introduces a voice search application in 2001. It becomes very popular because it becomes the first voice-detected application. Communication between people and technology has become very easy with this approach of Google.

- In 2002: Two main types of research are conducted in 2002 and they are as follows: Global Autonomous Language Exploitation and Effective Affordable Reusable (EARS) speech to text recognition.
- In 2007: After hiring some researchers in Google Company, a telephone-based directory service GOOGLE-411 her first effort at speech recognition came in 2007.
- In 2011: Apple works on our voice and launched SIRI which is faster, interact with your voice with an Apple device. As we know, now a day many most popular voice-command-based virtual assistants are in higher demand like our SIRI, ALEXA, GOOGLE HOME'S and many more.
- In 2017: Microsoft Researchers in 2017, a human parity milestone of transcribing conversational telephony was researched.

Table 1 shows the work progress of different authors in their research chapters.

NATURAL LANGUAGE PROCESSING (NLP)

Natural Language Processing (NLP)

Our best example of NLP is speech-to-text conversion which is an updated version of Deep Learning in which it can understand speech and react according to it as human beings do. The basic idea behind NLP is to feed the human language in the form of data for intelligent systems to consider and then utilize in various domains (Mittrapiyanuruk et al. 2000).

Text to speech and speech to text conversion means using NLP we are trying to do speech and text recognition techniques as shown in Figure 3. Our NLP can understand human language because it belongs to the field of Artificial Intelligence that gives them the ability to follow all instructions as humans do. (Rachakonda et al. 2021) Top MNC companies and start-up companies are putting more effort and millions of money into the NLP field. Everywhere the data scientist's are trying to understand the NLP domain and its process with excellent application. Most of the industries try to connect NLP directly in their technology (Humble and Mozelius 2019).

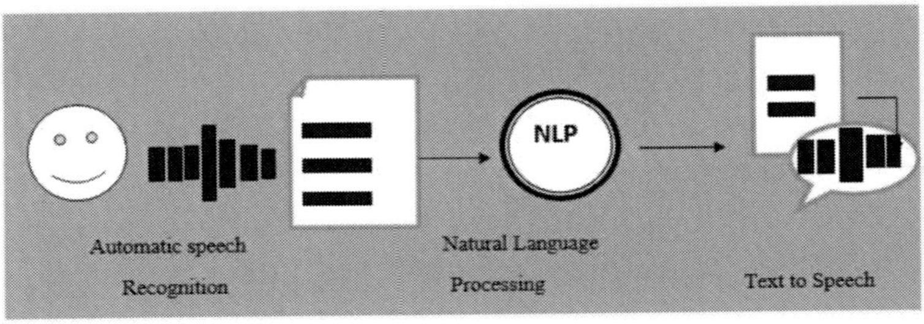

Figure 3. How to build specific automatic speech Recognition.

Applications of NLP- Speech to Text and Vice Versa

- Natural Language Processing has made it possible to entertain another important human behavior. Comprehension of language has made it possible to bring about all the transformational technologies. The basic examples of such are SIRI and ALEXA are more commercial applications and regular call center agents on a more operational scale.
- Using the deep learning algorithms, the NLP can do a lot with the unstructured data by finding patterns of sentiments, by doing data mining, and specific text slates within a block of text.
- Helping us out with the text-to-speech systems. For our view, we will focus on speech to text which will allow us to use audio as a primary source of data and then train our model through deep learning.

- Unique sounds that we make in a specific tone, voice, through our movement of lips and then tongue too. We have five senses and no one mentions a word recognition of people's voices.
- One commonly used Python text to speech conversion library is 'pyttsx3.' Unlike other libraries, it also works offline and is better with both Python 2 and 3. Everywhere used this technique like the film industry dubbing the movie, converting the male voice to female voice.
- VOICE BIOMETRICS: Interpretation algorithm works on voice. We use the previously stored voice messages in this technology so that we can produce the result of the current one.
- NEW SIRI TECHNOLOGY: This technology includes the sensor which performs the instruction given by the speaker and developed by a famous company APPLE MACINTOSH in their iPhones.
- DEVELOPED TOYS AND GAMES: Some voice-activated toys and games are available in today's market which manually follows the owner's commands.
- HOME AUTOMATION: To maintain proper security at home you should prefer to control signals and voice-activated alarms.

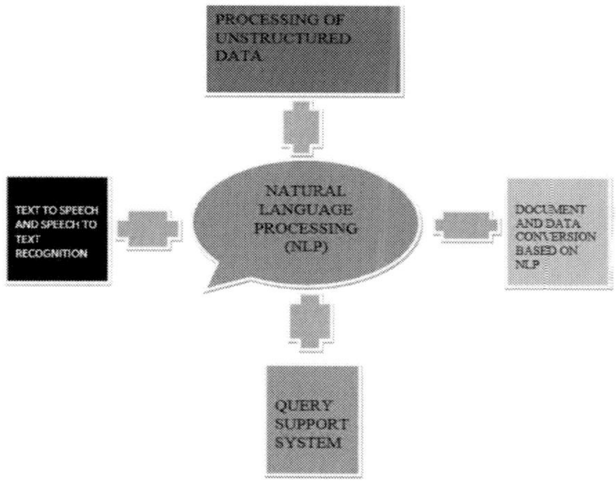

Figure 4. Architecture of Natural Language Processing (NLP).

UNSTRUCTURED DATA

We can define unstructured data as a type of information that is not pre-defined or data is not organized manner. As we know that Emails, messages, photos, videos, web pages, and so on are some unstructured business documents. “Unstructured data comprises the vast majority of data found in an organization, some estimates run as high as 80%” is said Merrill Lynch in 1998 (Qady and Abdelrahman 2008).

In unstructured data, we include various techniques like Data analytics, Data Mining, Natural Processing Language (NLP) to find different patterns or to interpret the information.One common framework is there for processing this information to extract meaningful information and to create structured data about the given document is the Unstructured Information Management Architecture (UIMA) standard (Adnan, Akbar, and Wang 2019).

Approaches in Natural Language Processing

To convert unstructured data into structured data within the text data and document you have to develop a specific computational workflow. To handle thousands or millions of data or those documents which are far away from manual approaches which need permit can be done by the specific computational workflow. In today’s world, these approaches are generally based on online Transaction Processing Systems (OLTP) or maybe on text cubes (Adnan, Akbar, and Wang 2019).

EXAMPLES OF UNSTRUCTURED DATA

In this column, we include some examples of unstructured data, or this data may be some video, audio, social media post, sensors, or maybe image files. (Adnan, Akbar, and Wang 2019)These data are following some well-defined timestamps, from and to concepts like in email which is also unstructured data. Internet of Things (IoT) adds machine to machine and sensor flowing out of it.

- Email: As we know that Email is unstructured data and cannot be parsed using analytics tools. But sometimes Email is also present in structured data so we can say our Emails as semi-structured data.
- Different Text files: These files include speed sheets, MS Word files, Email, Excel files, Presentation files, and so on.
- Social media and websites: Data from various social networking sites like Twitter, LinkedIn, Facebook, and some other websites like YouTube, Photo sharing sites, and Instagram.
- Mobile and communications data: Some communication methods are there like text messages, phone call recording, and so on.
- Social Media: On social video, many photos, videos, and images are posted.
- Scientific Surveys: Many survey reports like atmospheric data, oil and gas surveys, space exploitation, and scientific images. (Swamidason et al. 2020)
- Digital cameras used for surveillance: Some personal photos and videos we can get from digital surveillance.
- Image getting from Satellite: we get images of weather reports, landforms and Military movements send by satellite.

Three Use Cases for Unstructured Data

Here are a few examples where unstructured data is being used in analytics today: (Adnan, Akbar, and Wang 2019)

- Classifying image and sound: With the help of Deep Learning, we can easily recognize images and sounds. For example, a computer is designed in such a way that it can identify certain sounds that a motor is failing. This technology can also be used in automobiles and aviation.

- As input to predictive models: If you want to structure your unstructured data so the best way is to use Text analytics based on NLP and Machine learning. For example, to build a predictive model of customers so you can use call center notes to extract entities, sentiments, or themes and this information can be combined with other information to get the result.
- Chatbots in customer experience: Chatbots are there in the market but the new and developed chat boats are more in demand because they are having a better understanding of languages as well as more attractive. There is a great experience to become a customer of chatbots, based on who you are and what you want and you will be routed to the right representative to answer your queries.

Data Mining

Data Mining can be defined as the extraction of useful data from unstructured data and to use of various data patterns. Data mining is a very intelligent method and a result of the natural evolution of information technology. The use of data mining in unstructured is to ingextracting data out of it.

For Example, if we have an unstructured document like a letter of two or more parties. So our unstructured data mining technique would break down the letter into sub-parts for getting bits of information. And after the mining process is completed, it is then put in a format so that it can be recognized easily.

Challenges in Unstructured Data Mining

- Usability: For structure data to be usable, the business will have to come up with a way to locate and store data.
- Volume: The volume of unstructured data is growing at a rate of 60% per year which challenges both using and securing the data.
- Incompleteness: Incomplete data create uncertainties and they must be resolved during analysis.
- Quality: On a consumer level, people could be negatively impacted by companies that make a decision based on unstructured data. On an enterprise level, making a business decision based on inaccurate data could be extremely costly.
- Relevance: One way in which relevance comes into the picture is a lack of insight into the previous story of certain pieces of data.

QUERY SUPPORT SYSTEMS

A query is a system that is used to get information from the database. Particularly in Robust database systems, query system makes it easier to edit in large quantities of data and to perceive the trends at a high level (Sharma and Bhardwaj 2014).

Three Types of Search Queries

- Navigational search queries: for finding particular web pages and websites many users visited our Navigational search query system. For example, "Facebook" and "YouTube" are the viewed searches on Google, and they both are navigational queries. The navigational query has a much-focused goal i.e., users are very sure about their useful site and if you do not belong to their site or you're don't know about that site, you are not useful for the user. Google is the only site that clarifies this problem as a 'go query.' Some queries that appear to be navigational might not be. Suppose you type 'YOUTUBE' on Google it means you are looking for information related to their site as shown in Figure 5.

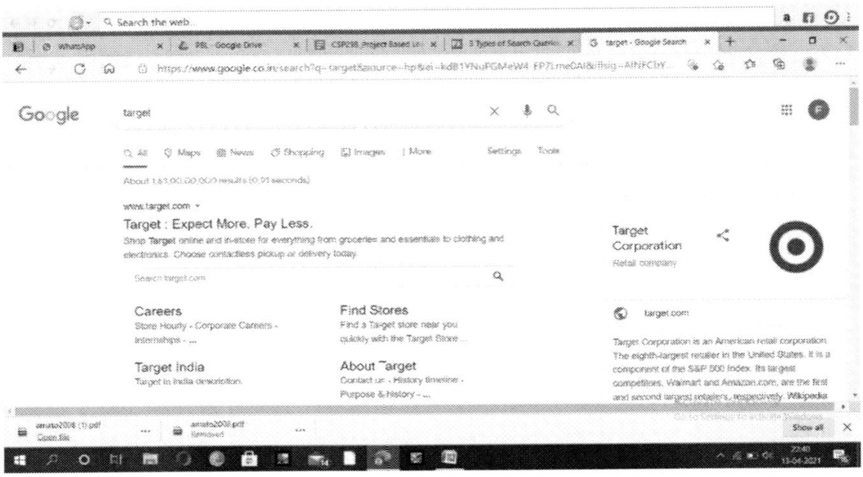

Figure 5. Navigational Search Query.

- Informational search queries: In an information query you can find a thousand relevant results for any information. When someone enters a query in Google or any other search engine- they are looking for entered name information and this happens only through an informational search query. They just do not want any specific site as shown in the navigational query system, they just want an answer to their question and this can be done by the informational search query. For example, Wikipedia gave a lot of information about the particular information, their history, their advantages, and uses, and so on. The main focus of this query is to prove yourself an authoritative source of information, become trustworthy, and don't want to misuse your personal information as shown in Figure 7.

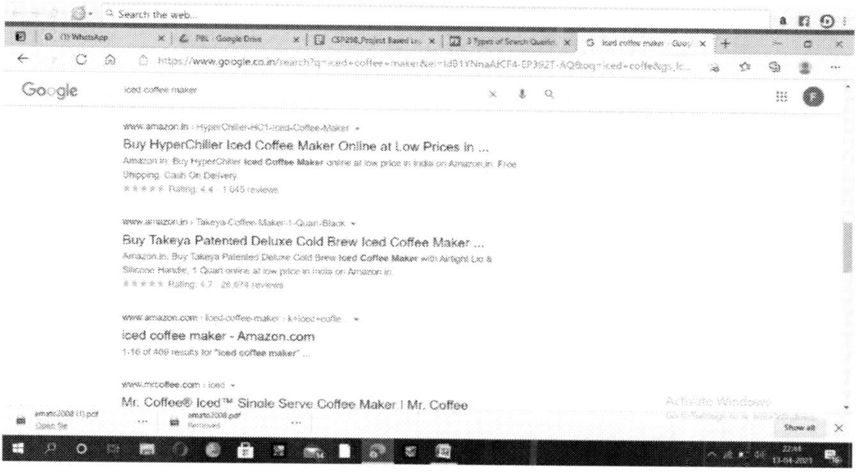

Figure 6. Informational search Queries.

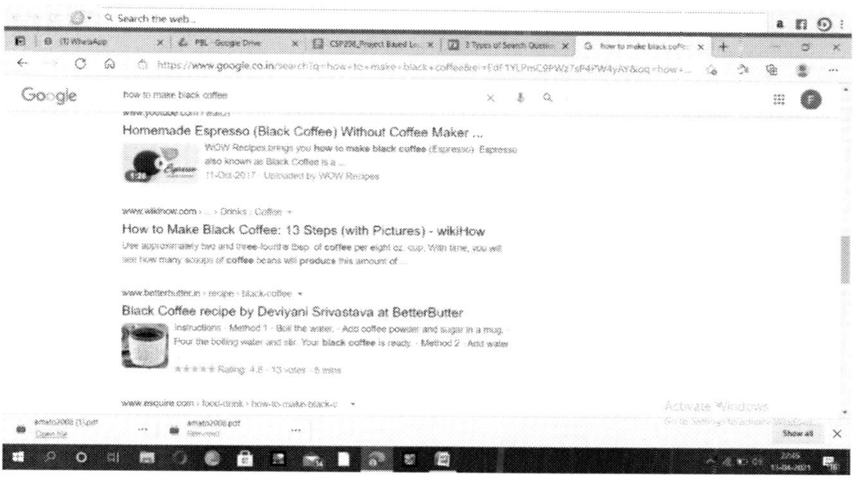

Figure 7. Transactional Search Queries.

- Transactional search queries: In this query system you have to complete your transaction by purchasing a particular product. This type of search query includes the exact product name and brand or includes "buy," "purchase," and "order." Vertical searches are a subset of a transactional search query and it represents the people who are interested to make a transaction in a specific company. To increase our sales percentage and in a cost-efficient way, you can go with 'AdWords' which is a good example for a transactional search query as shown in Figure 7.

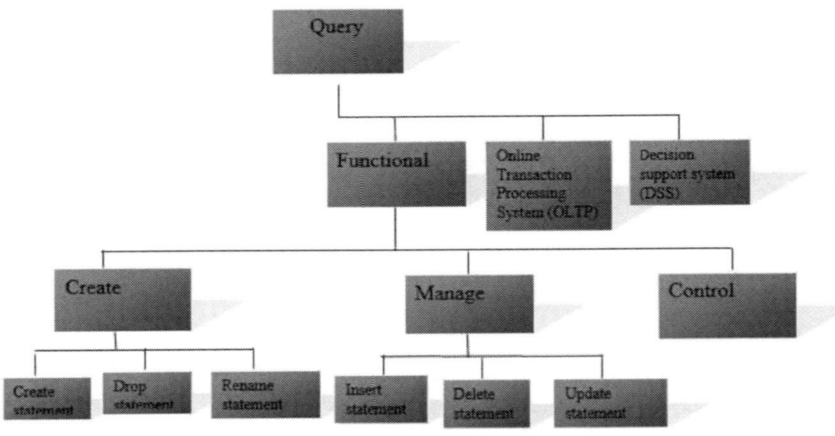

Figure 8. Different sections of Query support system. (Sharma and Bhardwaj 2014).

In Figure 8, we learned various sections of a query support system like the Functional part, the online transaction processing system (OLTP), and the Decision support system (DSS). And our Functional part is divided into Create, Manage and Control where we see we can create our query support system in various ways like by creating a statement, by using Drop statement and also using Rename statement. And in all these forms we just create statements in different forms. And also, we can manage the query support system by using the Insert statement, delete statement, and also by updating statement. As shown in Figure 7.

Online Transaction Processing System

OLTP is used for transaction-oriented applications and to facilitate typical information systems. OLTP has been used to refer to the requests of the user immediately. For example, ATM is used in the bank for commercial transaction processing applications as described in Figure 9.

It can also be used to update and insert in database management. The main aim of OLTP is to achieve speed, recoverability, concurrency in our transactions. OLTP application can be done by the combination of input messages, use of existing files, by processing and updating the data. OLTP can be achieved by the client-server system. If you want to increase your OLTP performance you have to avoid excessive use of clusters and indexes. As shown in figure 8 (Stanik et al. 2018).

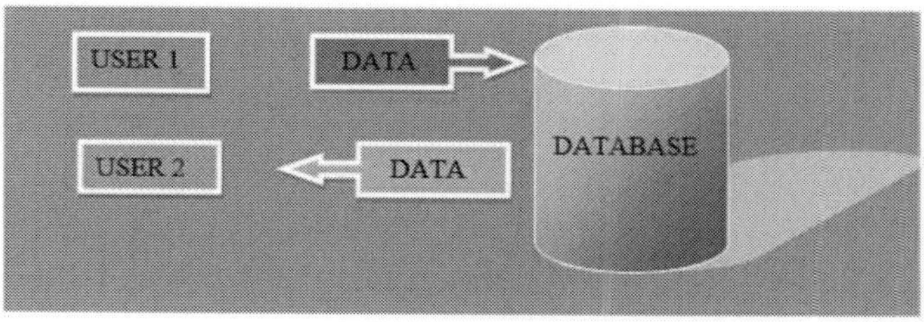

Figure 9. Transfer of data in OLTP.

Decision Support System (DSS)

A Decision Support System as described in Figure 10, can be defined as an effective way of using a computer to help decision-makers to solve unstructured data using various data and models.DSS has many forms and can be used in many different ways like focus on data, communication, or focus on models. The most important use of DSS is that they provide information that is very helpful in Decision-making processes. This system provides relevant schemes which solve the problem provided by the user. It is closely related to data mining and also manages the unstructured data and web pages. Web-based Decision support system and OLTP is mostly used Decision Support system in today's world. As shown in Figure 9 (Stanik et al. 2018).

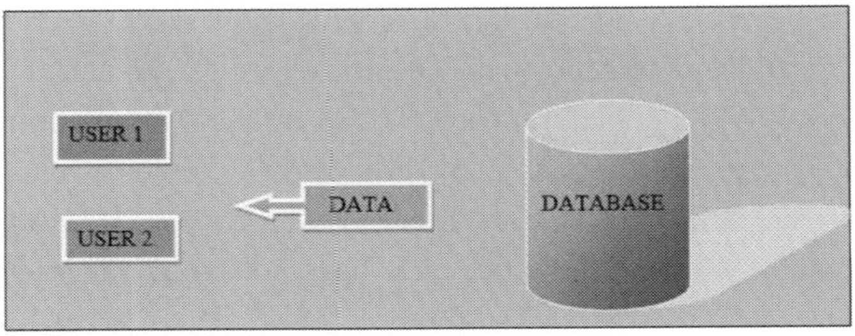

Figure 10. Transfer of data in DSS.

Documents and Data Conversion

Like a lot of document increases day by day so it is difficult for the business to organize and manage that data so data can be converted into digital format with the help of a data conversion service. Digitized data provides visibility, accessibility, and data security also (Qady and Abdelrahman 2008).

There are several file formats so you can view your data in many different formats. Converting the data makes it a better way to understand that data as well as derive new insight from it.

Different Types of File Format for Businesses

- DOC: This format is used in the format of Microsoft Word. It changes images, formats, tables, or any other forms of data. It is one of the famous file formats uses by many businesses for several reasons. It makes file editing easier, graphic-rich text, and so on(Sharma and Bhardwaj 2014).
- TXT: This is a file format used for a text file that can be created by word processing files. As compared to the DOC file this format is not flexible as it works only for text editing and does not support images or graphs. However, it secures our data and uses by many organizations.

- HTML: This file format is related to web addresses and web pages. Almost all word systems can use this format to edit the text into an HTML extension. This file can be viewed on a regular website.
- PPT: PowerPoint is a widely used application used by many students, teachers, businessmen, and organizations to represent their presentations and seminars. It supports many things like graphs, tables, text, images, animations, and video-audio, and so on (Sharma and Bhardwaj 2014).
- PDF: It is also the most popular file format used by many businesses. Adobe work on this extension to make our presentation more effective. It also supports 3D drawing, graphs, images, text, and more. PDF can make a big file into a smaller size so that we can share it easily.

Document Conversion Services

File and Document conversion services help us to improve our performance and efficiency. FREE data conversion services are also provided by many websites and we can also do online document conversion by using some extensions as mention below.

These extensions just convert your document into the format you need for your business line in Catalogs, reports, images, legal statements into the specific format as you need and in books also. Our FREE data conversion services are of high value in today's market (Qady and Abdelrahman 2008).

Many ways are there for Document Conversion Services such as:

- Auto CAD conversion
- Document conversion
- Standard Generalized Makeup Language
- GIF TO TGA conversion
- Book conversion service

- DWG TO JPG
- PSD TO XHTML
  - PDF to Word, Doc, MS Excel, HTML, XML format
  - Word to XML, HTML, PDF format
  - Scan images to electronic format
  - Graphic formatting

Word Conversion Services:

- For a quick and easy way of converting your files into word, the pictures in them so you should use our given word conversion files services which is suitable for you at a point.
- As compared to other services you have only convert the important files into word files without giving some payments but in our word, conversion services your original formatting is there, your tables, images, graphs, and diagram all are there without any changes.

We can convert the following Format into Word Documents: (Qady and Abdelrahman 2008)

- HTML
- PDF
- Image Extraction and Scan reports
- PowerPoint Presentation
- Microsoft Excel
- Chapter and Document
- E-book services
- Text Conversion
- Use of XML.

Conclusion

Our chapter is based on NLP i.e., Natural Language Processing and its various uses like Text to speech and speech to text conversion, Processing of Unstructured Data, Document and Data conversion, Query support system, and so on. We mainly focused on how we can achieve above mention mechanism using NLP. And we conclude how we convert both text and speech into each other, various steps should be done like speech recognition, convert it into an audio file, and so on. We can also do some coding to achieve our goal. We can understand the features of NLP by seeing the architecture of NLP which is subdivided into Document and Data conversion, Query support system, unstructured Data, and so on. We can learn various query support systems and how we can get information about a particular product, how to purchase it. Different word file conversion and other techniques are given to convert our data and documents.

In the end, we reach a point that our texting system which includes Unstructured data, Query support systems, Document, and data conversion all are based on NLP of to achieve all these things we have to study a lot about NLP.

References

Adnan, Kiran, Rehan Akbar, and Khor Siak Wang. 2019. "Information Extraction from Multifaceted Unstructured Big Data." *International Journal of Recent Technology and Engineering (IJRTE)* 8: 1398–1404.

Bakiri, Ghulum. 1991. "Converting English Text to Speech: A Machine Learning Approach."

Bandhu, Reeta, Nikhil Kumar Singh, and Betawar Shashank Sanjay. 2019. "Offline Speech Recognition on Android Device Based on Supervised Learning." *International Journal of Advance Research. Ideas and Innovations in Technology* 5 (2): 985–87.

Humble, Niklas, and Peter Mozelius. 2019. "Artificial Intelligence in Education—A Promise, a Threat or a Hype." In *Proceedings of the European Conference on the Impact of Artificial Intelligence and Robotics*, 149–56.

Ifeanyi, Nwakanma, Oluigbo Ikenna, and Okpala Izunna. 2014. "Text--To--Speech Synthesis (TTS)." *International Journal of Research in Information Technology* 2 (5).

Khilari, Prachi, and V P Bhope. 2015. "Implementation of Speech to Text Conversion." *International Journal of Innovative Research in Science, Engineering and Technology* 4 (7): 6441–50.

Mahanta, Deepshikha, Bidisha Sharma, Priyankoo Sarmah, and S R Mahadeva Prasanna. 2016. "Text to Speech Synthesis System in Indian English." In *2016 IEEE Region 10 Conference (TENCON)*, 2614–18.

Mittrapiyanuruk, Pradit, Chatchawarn Hansakunbuntheung, Virongrong Tesprasit, and Virach Sornlertlamvanich. 2000. "Issues in Thai Text-to-Speech Synthesis: The NECTEC Approach." *NECTEC Technical Journal* 2 (7): 36–47.

Prasad, Vijay. 2015. "Voice Recognition System: Speech-to-Text." *Journal of Applied and Fundamental Sciences* 1 (2): 191.

Qady, Al, and Mohammed Abdelrahman. 2008. *Concept Relation Extraction Using Natural Language Processing: The CRISP Technique.*

Sharma, Komal, and Ankur Bhardwaj. 2014. "Types of Queries in Database System." *International Journal of Computer Applications and Information Technology* 7 (2): 149–52.

Shih, Chilin, and Richard Sproat. 1996. "Issues in Text-to-Speech Conversion for Mandarin." In *International Journal of Computational Linguistics & Chinese Language Processing, Volume 1, Number 1, August 1996*, 37–86.

Stanik, Christoph, Lloyd Montgomery, Daniel Martens, Davide Fucci, and Walid Maalej. 2018. "A Simple NLP-Based Approach to Support Onboarding and Retention in Open Source Communities." In

2018 IEEE International Conference on Software Maintenance and Evolution (ICSME), 172–82.

Swamidason, Iwin Thanakumar Joseph, Sravanthi Tatiparthi, V M Arul Xavier, and C S C Devadass. 2020. "Exploration of Diverse Intelligent Approaches in Speech Recognition Systems." *International Journal of Speech Technology*, 1–10.

Trivedi, Ayushi, Navya Pant, Pinal Shah, Simran Sonik, and Supriya Agrawal. 2018. "Speech to Text and Text to Speech Recognition Systems-Areview." *IOSR Journal of Computer Engineering* 20 (2): 39.

Rachakonda Hrithik Sagar, Abhishek Bingi, Aashray Pola, Krishna Sai Raj Goud, Tuiba Ashraf, Subrata Sahana. 2021. "Malignant Skin Cancer Detection Using Convolutional Neural Networking." *International Journal of Engineering Science & Technology* V06.I05: 001.

In: Intelligent Information Retrieval … ISBN: 978-1-68507-301-5
Editors: Parma Nand et al. © 2021 Nova Science Publishers, Inc.

Chapter 10

STORING AND MAINTAINING THE SMART HEALTHCARE IN IOT ENVIRONMENT

N. Ambika**, PhD
Department of Computer Applications,
Sivananda Sarma Memorial RV College,
Bangalore, India

ABSTRACT

IoT device use in healthcare has helped physicians to analyze the condition of the patient. The monitoring can happen by the doctors without being on the hospital premises. These devices are a great help in managing the doings. IoT device use in healthcare has helped the physicians to analyze the condition of the patient staying at a long distance. The previous work proposes a keen medical services framework in an IoT climate. It can screen a patient's essential health signal as the room condition. The wired sensors gather information from the patient's body. It employs an ESP32 module and ships off the entryway worker. Five sensors catch the information from the clinic climate sensors. They include a heartbeat sensor, internal heat level sensor, room-temperature sensor, CO sensor, and CO_2 sensor. The

* Corresponding Author's E-mail: Ambika.nagaraj76@gmail.com.

mistake level is inside a specific breaking point for each case. The state of the patients is at the entrance to clinical staff. It can measure and examine the current circumstance of the patients. The proposal aims to store the measured values. These stored quantities can help doctors suggest future treatment for the patient. The proposal increases availability by 33.55% compared with the previous contribution.

Keywords: IoT, healthcare, ThingSpeak

INTRODUCTION

The Internet of Things (Whitmore, Agarwal and Da Xu 2015) (Nagaraj 2021) is a recognizable possible answer for lightening factors on medical care frameworks. The exploration checks patients with definite conditions, such as diabetes sickness. The various advantages are far-off wellbeing checking. The new scientists have recognized the capability of the Internet of Things (Mehdi Khosrow-Pour 2020) as an answer for medical care. It is a previously mentioned field that shows up immensely extraordinary to medical care. The examination led inside them confirms the believability of an IoT-based medical care framework. Existing frameworks in different domains have demonstrated that distant checking of items with information assortment and detailing is feasible. IoT medical services frameworks (N. Ambika, 2020) are for explicit purposes, including recovery, diabetes the executives, helps encompassing living for adults, and then some.

The significant advancements for the ideal medical services framework are sensor discovery, network modernization, and information preparing innovation. Information preparation incorporates computerized imaging preparing, symptomatic programming, and electronic wellbeing record frameworks. Ongoing investigations in the IoT have offered a large number of conceivable outcomes. Its standards are applicable to improve the nature of care, the availability, and save the expense. The IoT gives attention to its patients in far-off areas. It checks frameworks that convey a nonstop significant information stream for better choices in acknowledged miniature remote physiological sensors to set up versatile medical care frameworks in their examination. It utilizes remote physiological sensors joined with intelligent cell phones. It executes patients concentrated checking, crisis care, following, investigation, analysis, caution triggering, locating, and joint effort with clinical staff. It is the case that IoT sensor procedure is applied to assemble patient information to set up a versatile medical care framework. In extended the idea of IoT to a few segments in a medical services framework, he proposed the IoT stage for medical services as a suitable self-administration model for persistent sicknesses like heftiness, hypertension, and diabetes.

Radio Frequency Identification, sensors, and portable addresses are three of the most promising advances. It empowers the execution of medical services frameworks. RFID (Jia et al. 2012) is low-power innovation comprising latent or potentially battery-helped aloof gadgets named labels, which can send information when controlled by the electromagnetic field produced by an investigator named peruser. Since inactive RFID labels do not need a wellspring of energy to work, their lifetime estimates in many years, along these lines making the RFID innovation well fit in an assortment of utilization situations, including medical care. There is new accessibility of UHF RFID labels with expanded capacities. Indeed, RFID-based detecting in medical care empowers zero-power, ease, and simple to execute checking and transmitting patient physiological boundaries. In any case, the fundamental disadvantage of RFID labels originates from working exclusively under the peruser inclusion district.

Such an angle restricts the utilization of UHF RFID innovation to protest proof and checking inside tiny territories.

Keen health devices allow you naturally to log your clinical information through Bluetooth entitled gadgets. It observes your health by putting away, breaking down, and sharing your clinical records. It likewise prompts you on tips and administrations dependent on your health examination. It additionally gives you alarms and messages about your health hazards. It empowers you to screen the reports. It has the alternative interfacing with different health specialist co-ops like pharma, labs, home consideration, and teleconsulting. Cooey is the health checking IoT estage. It helps the suppliers in gathering, putting away, and dissecting crude clinical information. It gives alarms of vital signs to patients already. It allows you to pick and redo your customized administrations dependent on your health condition. For clients, it is health a board application with customized administrations. It is an answer for the persistent health of the executives. No other item and application can give a last-mile association of a patient with his health specialists. Cooey can interconnect and offer centered types of assistance to its clients.

The work proposes a keen medical services framework (Islam, Rahaman, and Islam 2020) in IoT environment. It can screen a patient's essential health signal. The wired sensors gather information from the patient's body. It employs an ESP32 module and ships off the entryway worker. For the web UI, ThingSpeak aid in for the graphical translation, and show of gathered outcomes. ThingSpeak shows the current status and cycle of exchanges. The HTTP convention gives a simple network to the correspondence between a Wi-Fi module and the webserver. Five sensors catch the information from the clinic climate sensors. They include a heartbeat, internal heat level, room-temperature sensor, CO, and CO_2 sensor. The mistake level is at a specific breaking point. The state of the patients is at the entrance of the clinical staff. It can measure and examine the current circumstance of the patients.

The work compares with previous work. The first part of the care cloud (Shakil et al. 2020) is chargeable for the management of patients report and alternative data. It has trio layers. The supplier tier divides into body and security levels. The biometric identification agent acts at the protection level. The shopper tier provides associate degree interaction between the cloud and its users. The protection and resource provisioning is successively handled by the two parts of the health service supplier level severally.

The storage and its management area unit is the responsibility of the info center level. The Health Information Management System is chargeable for the management, storage, and retrieval of the information. The workers and patients register within the healthcare center area unit. They give their signature samples victimization either the signature capturing device or their smartphones that area unit put in with the signature capturing package. It captures the user's signature. The standard of the given signature checks victimization SigQuality checker package. The performance of this package confirms the recorded signature samples. It matches up to the standard standards needed for authentication. The options of the samples area unit extracted and area unit keep within the care cloud. The practitioner will be able to view the data after the update. The suggestion enables modification and updating of data. It also allows viewing the data with only the user credentials.

The biometry (N. Ambika 2020) of the personnel and patient extraction generates the individual hash value. It is on the server. Whenever the worker examines the patient, the worker demonstrates himself by giving the biometry and location details. The hash value for identical is generated and cross-verified with the information hold on the server. On positive confirmation, the personnel area unit was allowed to update the analysis outline of the patient. The identical is updated. This value is concatenated with the information and submitted to the server. Comparing this work to the suggestion location information is necessary. The proposal aims to view the records after authenticating with either of their credentials. The user (doctor/patient) will be able to view the data related to them. To modify or update them, both the credentials become necessary.

The suggestion stores the data and provides a management method where only legitimate users can see the records. The procedure commences with the registration stage, where the doctor and the patient credentials are collected. It generates the hash content using credentials. This substance acts as an authenticator in different values. The doctor or the patient has access to view the details fed earlier using their credentials. To modify and update details, the details of doctor and sick are essential. The data transmitted after authentication also generates a hash value to adapt reliability in the system. It detects any modification in the previously stored data at an earlier stage. It helps in making appropriate decisions. The proposal increases availability by 33.55% compared with the previous contribution.

The literature survey follows the introduction section in segment two. The third division commences with the description of the previous work and follows with the narration of the present proposal. The next segment analyses the work by simulating it. The chapter concludes in division fifth division.

LITERATURE SURVEY

The section talks about various contributions to the domain.

The work proposes a medical framework (Islam, Rahaman, and Islam 2020). It can screen a patient's essential health signal as the room condition. The wired sensors gather information from the patient's body. It employs an ESP32 module and ships off the entryway worker. For the web UI, ThingSpeak aid in for the graphical translation, and show of gathered outcomes. ThingSpeak shows the current status and cycle of exchanges. The HTTP convention gives a simple network to the correspondence between a Wi-Fi module and the webserver. Five sensors catch the information from the clinic climate sensors. They include a heartbeat sensor, internal heat level sensor, room-temperature sensor, CO sensor, and CO_2 sensor. The mistake level is a specific breaking point. The state of the patients is at the entrance to clinical staff. It can measure and examine the current circumstance of the patients.

It is definite health observing framework (Gupta et al. 2016). It is sufficiently keen to screen the patient utilizing IoT. It gathers the status data through these frameworks. It incorporates the patient's pulse, circulatory strain, and ECG and sends a crisis alarm to the primary care physician with his current status and clinical data. It would help the specialist to screen his patient from any place and to the patient to send his health status straightforwardly without visiting the emergency clinic. The model conveys to different emergency clinics and clinical organizations. The framework utilizes intelligent sensors that create crude information data gathered from every sensor and send it to a data set worker. The information can be additionally dissected and measurably kept up to be utilized by clinical specialists. Keeping an information base worker is an unquestionable requirement so that there is even track of past clinical records of the patient giving superior and improved inspecting.

It has three (Catarinucci et al. 2015) primary parts. SHS expects a few 6LR are sent to the medical clinic to gather information from the climate, like temperature, pressure, and surrounding light conditions. Notwithstanding the detecting abilities, the principle capacity of 6LRR hubs, all things being equal, is to follow patients, nursing staff, and biomedical gadgets marked with RFID Gen2 tags. The sensed information is intermittently signed on the client memory of the RFID Gen2 tag, accordingly permitting 6LRR hubs sent in the climate to recover and convey them to the IoT Smart Gateway. It is associated, from one perspective, straightforwardly with the HSN and, then again, with the Internet through a Local Area Network (LAN). The specialists prepare with a cell phone associated with a versatile RFID Gen2 peruser. It is running a modified application named Medical App. The specialists can connect straightforwardly with the HT hub worn by the patient. He checks his physiological boundaries by perusing the latest data put away into the client memory of the RFID Gen2 tag or verifiable data put away into the Control data set. The Medical App permits specialists likewise to refresh the memory content with data to remind.

The ECG checking hub (Yang et al. 2016) gathers information from the human skin and sends this learning to the passageway through a remote channel. The sensor module is the observing hub and is liable for accumulating ECG information from the human body. WITH the AD8232 ECG sensor and fringe circuits, frail ECG signs distinguish with good exactness. The regulator module measures the accumulated ECG signal and sends them to the Wi-Fi module. All the sign handling capacities carry out in an elite Microcontroller Unit. It is in signal handling applications due to its incredible equipment, e.g., the 32-bit

ARM CortexM3 miniature regulator working at 72 MHz, a Flash memory up to 512 Kbytes, and a broad scope of improved input/output and peripherals associated employing two APB means of transport.

The optical preparing center point (Khan et al. 2020) gets visual data from visual sensors as a video outline in the savvy medical care observation organizations, prompting critical measures. The transportation of all video in real-time is ridiculous because of the more extensive territory (distance) between the base station and visual handling center due to data transmission as the energy impediments of WMSNs. It presents and dissects the recommended cosine change-based turbulent grouping attributes. It is like an encryption interaction in a shrewd medical care IoT framework that separates from the visual sensor stream. The proposed calculation has two primary parts. The principal division plans to utilize the most recent cosine change-based turbulent succession to produce PRNG suitable for our proposed picture encryption. The subsequent one intends to perform three rounds of disarray. The CTC succession has shortcomings in fragile turmoil and frail powerful inclinations. The blended strategy rearranges the mayhem construction of both two seed succession maps effectively. The cosine change shows exceptionally muddled non-linearity.

Five parts of IoT healthcare structure (Jeong, Han, and You 2016) is a roundabout framework. The sensor gathers information and goes to the subsequent stage. It is a keen organization to speak with the framework. Sending a message through the organization is put away at distributed computing which is the third segment. The information undergoes examination for reliable choice in the fourth segment enormous knowledge examination. After choosing a legitimate outcome of information, refined information ships off to a savvy clinic. It educates the processed data to medical services experts. The intelligent clinic makes moves for fitting analysis and treatment. The information assortment highlight comprises IoT-driven sensors to gather constant observing information from sensors. Sensor innovation accomplishes progress to deal with information in bio optic sensors. It also includes EEG biotelemetry, ECG sensors. It is a model for executing omnipresent, on-request admittance to a shared pool of configurable processing environments. The information assortment comprises IoT-driven sensors to gather continuous observing information from intelligent sensors. The data assembled from the sensors ought to be accessible in the distributed computing conditions to be overseen and worked appropriately. Subsequently, an essential issue of programming controls the data from the sensor's distantly disseminated data. Cloud is on-request processing and is a sort of Internet-based figuring condition that gives shared preparing gadgets and information to PCs. The information investigation module performs by AI. AI is the study of creating PCs to act without being unequivocally programmed. The interface and the board module give an interface for the approved workforce. It includes specialists, insurance agencies and oversees clinical records. Some instances are the examined information of patients and the past clinical history. The perception of information for patient data is a significant idea of information practice to analyze and treat.

It is a novel Secure De-copied Data Scattering plan for Smart Healthcare IoT (Ullah et al. 2018) where the FoG worker is at the edge. It decreases delays in sending medical services information from sensors to focal stores in the cloud. It thinks about numerous gatherings of patients with different sensors on their bodies. Every individual has a gatherer hub on his body that is associated with the cell phone. Information de-duplication is on the gatherer hub. The Data collection is at the cell phone level and sinks level. The patient information extricates so that every patients' readings are put away in a focal store in the cloud. These records are made available online to specialists and clinic staff for assistance. It utilizes a versatile piecing calculation at the information sink. It secures message transmission from a brilliant medical care gadget to the gatherer. It advances to the FoG worker employing sink hub for preparing and capacity.

In medical care (Zhu et al. 2019), clinical information is caught by sensors and sent to the cloud worker to deal with savvy examination through various kinds of IoT organizations. The radio range utilization of these organizations shifts from 3G/4G, WIFI to 5G, LPWAN, and

LPLAN. Distinctive correspondence conventions application is dependent on the clinical application necessities. These expanded radio ranges permit a lot simpler and less expensive worldwide broadband development of shrewd medical services. Medical care is an information concentrated area where clinical information is gathered, put away, and got to consistently. A user can set their objectives. As indicated by these objectives, the medical care suppliers will plan a related arrangement for every client. Sensors record the client's execution of the plan and report the record to medical care experts. The medical services advisors can change the arrangement, and it is time-dependent. The client can likewise give input to the medical care specialists to help redo the organization. Therefore, clients can take self-sufficient activities on the health of the executives.

The study (Alhussein et al. 2018) proposes a programmed and progressed technique for EEG-based seizure location. It is observing a segment of the intellectual medical services IoT system. They use scalp EEG, which is recorded by EEG sensors, as the info signal. The framework utilizes other medical services. Intelligent sensors record the mental and physiological signs and communicate them to the cloud employing the Internet. Aside from EEG, these signs incorporate patients' developments, motions, and facial articulations to decide their state. The intellectual framework settles on an ongoing choice on the exercises. The clinical consideration and administrations are dependent on their status. They decide on sending the information to the profound learning module. Assuming the intellectual framework accepts that a patient has a seizure, this framework settles to illuminate different partners. It sends the EEG information to the profound learning module. Signal handling and seizure identification happen in the cloud are delegated seizure or non-seizure with a likelihood score. The sent outcomes to clinical professionals or different partners can screen the patients. It settles on the fitting choices to help the patient. EEG signals have a low sign-to-commotion proportion and are touchy to outer and inward clamors. It is a novel profound learning model. It is a convolution neural organization and stacked auto-encoder. The system removes highlights. The stacked auto-encoder improves the subject-explicit highlights and exactness.

The model (BK and Muralidhara 2015)comprises PIC18F46K22 Microcontroller, Temperature sensor, Pulse Oximeter Sensor, Liquid Crystal Display, GSM MODEM, Piezo Electric Buzzer, Wi-Fi Module, Max232, GSM Modem, Regulated Power Supply. The PIC18F46K22 Microcontroller gathers the knowledge from the sensors and sends the information through Wi-Fi Protocol. The Protected information sent can be gotten to whenever by the specialists by composing the relating novel. The IP address is an Internet Browser toward the end-client gadget. It associates with GSM Modem to give data to the specialist/guardian. It reacts when the pulse is more prominent than 90 or under 60. It also responds when the temperature is fewer than 20 or more than 35. The signal turns on and cautions the overseer. LCD associates with a microcontroller to show the exchange interaction and medical services information. The UI's HTML page will consequently revive at regular intervals. The health status is persistently shipped off the specialist.

The Remote Health Monitoring System (Banka, Madan, and Saranya 2018) works on Raspberry pi. Raspberry Pi is an installment card-sized single-board microcontroller that upgrades essential software engineering instruction in universities and agricultural countries. The framework intends to constantly screen imperative boundaries.

The pulse, circulatory strain, and internal heat level are some of the examples. The data is put away on a cloud worker information base and shown through an online site or versatile application by an approved workforce. It refreshes the information on the web and sends an alarm to the specialists for anomaly detection. It anticipates the illness of the patient. The previous utilizes the MySQL DB module to connect Raspberry pi. The natural information from different IoT gadgets is gotten and put away on the worker. These gadgets incorporate sensors like temperature sensors, vibration sensors, BP sensors, and beat sensors. The information mining procedures anticipate the sort and nature of the infection or the issues the framework plans. Utilizing computerized reasoning can additionally ad-lib the framework by making it more astute.

The proposed framework (Budida and Mangrulkar 2017) intends to cover from start to finish. It is an efficient and creative application. It has two structure blocks. The primary capacity of the first building block is to accumulate all tactile information that identifies with the checking of the patients. The subsequent square capacity stores and interacts with the system. It is data where the specialists get fitness reports following the instance of the observed patients. The framework comprises a health checking framework that is sufficiently smart to screen the patient's wellness naturally utilizing IoT. It would assist the specialists with observing patient's reports from any place and whenever. The framework uses sensors that create crude information data gathered from every sensor. It sends it to an information worker where the information undergoes investigation.

The association between the various components is about the accompanying design of the framework (Naik and Sudarshan 2019). This framework has two sections- Equipment and programming. In the equipment, the unit has transmitters and recipients. The product unit incorporates programming dialects like Python, MATLAB. Each sensor value is put away in the worker and showed late qualities. The specialist may see the patient's information along with their comparing login subtleties. A specialist can see the patient's authentic documents and recommends changes in medications and remedies. Unique IDs and passwords for patients can see their records. The framework centers on the patient's illness. The wellness edge and gets the ideal outcome. A specialist consistently investigates the patient's ailment utilizing some fundamental boundaries.

The proposed infant checking system (Hussain et al. 2019) has control graphs for intelligent homes and nurseries. Contribution to the type of video outlines from the RPi with the appended camera fixed over the infant bed. The video outlines pass to the movement discovery where two unique strategies are applied exclusively. Their outcomes coordinate to accomplish better precision. It yields a twofold picture where the white pixels address the movement of the infant. The parallel picture figures by a controlled outline development system to draw a point on the graph. The control graph is for an entire stretch check for strange conduct. It sets apart as strange. The alarm produces if most of the focuses cross the upper or lower limit in a single span. The watchmen or guardians receive the created alert for snappy activities. It sees the present status of the child through live streaming. The equipment arrangement contains an RPi with a camera fixed over the bed of the child. RPi has a remote sensor that is associated with the isolated organization in the intelligent home. The arrangement is in nurseries where an organization of RPi's catches video information from various children. The general preparation done is preposterous. The camera connected to the RPi can be a night vision camera working in both light and dim situations.

The medical care framework (Mohapatra, Mohanty, and Mohanty 2019) is astute in screening the essential fitness boundaries of patients. It uses IoT and the cloud. It gathers the status of the patient's pulse and temperature. It sends a crisis notice to the primary care physician. It would assist the specialist by observing the patient. The pulse sensor and the temperature sensor are associated with an Arduino DIY board. The wellbeing boundaries estimated are communicated to the cloud. The cloud innovation stores, measures, and breaks down a gigantic measurement of medical services information from patients across various topographical zones. The cell phone is associated with the proposed framework with the assistance of a Wi-Fi association. The specialist's cell phone or PC gathers the wellbeing information of a specific patient. The specialist suggests appropriate medical services for the situation of a medical issue. It prompts a more brilliant medical care board framework. For the most part, the IoT framework includes the distinguishing layer, the vehicle layer, and the application layer. The sensors assume a significant in the recognizing layer. The vehicle layer proliferates data caught by the sensors. The interface between cloud design and the IoT framework moves the knowledge to the cloud. The application layer is the place where we can access the boundaries from the web.

The work (Gong et al. 2015) proposes two modules to ensure the security and protection of knowledge. Initially, a disarray framework created upsets learning before the meeting of the worker. Second, message scrambles in the strategy of Internet transmission. For this situation, regardless of whether an aggressor got the encoded or mixed information. The person interprets them to plaintext. The aggressor cannot acquire genuine information by paying off, coercing the medical attendants, specialists. The calculation the authors proposed guarantees the accuracy of the input information from the worker without the reason of accomplishing the legitimate information.

The HealthFog model (Tuli et al. 2020) is an IoT-based fog-empowered cloud figuring model. It is a medical service that deals with the information of heart patients. It analyses the wellbeing status to distinguish coronary illness seriousness. The model incorporates assorted equipment instruments through programming segments and permits organized and consistent start to finish joining of Edge and Fog-Cloud for the quick and exact conveyance of results. Three distinct sorts of sensors establish this segment. Clinical sensors incorporate Electro Cardio Gram sensor, Electro Encephalo Gram sensor, Electro MyoGraphy sensor, oxygen level sensor, temperature sensor, breath rate sensor, and glucose level sensor. This part detects the information from the heart quiet and moves it to associated door gadgets. There are three distinct sorts of Gateway gadgets, which are going about as mist gadgets to gather detected information from various sensors forward this information to Worker hubs for additional preparation. The edges include the gateway, broker, and worker nodes. They are available in the same Local Area Network. The Resource Manager programming segment dwells in the broker node. The Gateway Broker Job demands a Labourer Cloud way gadgets send work demands to it. The assertion results got from the Resource Manager and the Gateway gadget. It educates it where to send the information. The Worker hubs intermittently send heartbeat parcels to the broker to show that they are alive. The bundles incorporate burden data used by the Resource Manager for load adjusting.

The IoT components (Salahuddin et al. 2018) incorporate intelligent sensors of various sizes and types. It can screen organic, substance, and actual boundaries, cycle and record crude tactile information. Handsets on the sensors empower correspondence with base stations through a remote interface. The more remarkable base stations go about as information aggregators, sink hubs, entryways to the Internet, and cloud or IoT passages for medical care applications and administrations. The IoT passages defeat the heterogeneity in gadgets and organization conventions and empower availability. The sensors locally measure the individual sensor estimations and figure the choice for a rule. The crude tangible information is prepared locally at the sensor. For example, a pulse dependent on electric voltage estimated by the ECG sensor sends to the ECG sensor entryway. The PPG sensor door gathers the stream rate and sends the data to the IoT entryway. The cardiovascular component of the patient accumulates and handles to medical care workers in the cloud. The information investigation and answers to approved medical care suppliers and workforce are available on their cell phones. The crude tangible information sends to sensor network entryways. It handles data and communicated it to the IoT door for logging and revealing.

The physiological boundaries (Bansal and Gandhi 2018) gather by different sensors put on the individual's body. The sensors can be ECG, EMG, EOG, and Blood Pressure. The information obtained from the individual is shipped off the IoT-based sheets like Arduino, Raspberry Pi, Intel Galileo. These sheets can make the medical services applications more open as they are intuitive articles. The sheets handle the information, and the message ships off to the specialist. If the individual is in a crisis, he can get input from the specialist.

Information is a combination design for a Smart Healthcare biological system (Dautov, Distefano, and Buyya 2019)recognized by coordinating with IoT framework abilities inside medical care associations with the current information combination models. The three-level information combination model orders IoT preparing components in matching and sending the low level into edge gadgets, the medium one into correspondence and handling units, or potentially the high one into far-off server farms. Low-level knowledge combination should occur on objects, which gather information coming from edge devices using doors or shrewd gadgets themselves. Center-level information combination alludes to perform more examination over data pushed from a more extensive organization of gadgets. It means to identify potential infection episodes by planning qualities from bed sensor gadgets to actual areas. These are positioned gadgets. It coordinates and deals with the staff all the more effectively. Undeniable level information combination alludes to the most elevated level of information combination, which gives a worldwide perspective overall oversaw arrangement of edge gadgets and systems administration hubs. It includes the preparation of information. It executes in a far-off data center or a Cloud. HDF gathers information from all clinics inside a city and performs information combinations over the metropolitan zone.

The proposed Gray Filter Bayesian Convolution Neural Network (Patan et al. 2020) is shrewd wellbeing care contributing towards clinical information examination. It illustrates computational productive wellbeing observing and conveyance data in a period for keen society. The technique comprises two terms. The assignment stays in gathering patient wellbeing knowledge for hearth observation of brilliant IoT gadgets. The information aggregated through savvy IoT gadgets in actual space communicates for additional investigation utilizing cloud specialist co-ops that use a distributed computing climate. The data is pre-handled with the assistance of dim sifting relies upon the gathered increasing activity. The pre-prepared highlights, Bayesian Logistic Sigmoid activation methods are applied to distinguish ideal human action. With this caught human action volume arrangement, softmax work exacts characterization dependent on the maximum pooling capacity.

Multimodal signal (Amin et al. 2019) obtaining is helped out through IoT sensors. The neighborhood comprises low-range specialized gadgets. This layer sends the gained signals from the smart IoT sensor and devices to the facilitating layer. The facilitating layer has various kinds of intelligent gadgets, such as media mobiles or PCs. It can store and send signals. The device sends the information got from the brilliant gadgets to the cloud unit. The WAN layer utilizes progressed correspondence organizations, like Wi-Fi, 4G, or 5G, to send information progressively to the cloud. The cloud chief in the cloud layer verifies the patient's information and sends them to the intellectual motor for preparation. IoT sensors comprise wearable and fixed sensors that can quantify clinical signs, for example, internal heat level, heartbeat, pulse, voice, outward appearances, body development, and EEG. A portion of these sensors is in the patient's environmental factors. These gadgets can speak with different devices utilizing IoT. The LAN comprises short-range correspondence conventions like Bluetooth, LoWPAN, and Zigbee. The facilitating layer has savvy gadgets, like media cell phones, tablets, and individual computerized associates. These gadgets store information locally and have committed projects for straightforward calculations on the got signals.

Information uses the WAN layer to move to the cloud handling unit. The cloud layer comprises a cloud supervisor, an intellectual motor, and a profound learning worker. The cloud supervisor is liable for the information stream. It carries out all the security conventions to check the personality of all brilliant city partners. After understanding verification, the intellectual motorcycles the information and decides the condition of the patient. It settles on choices and imparts EEG signs to the committed profound learning worker for EEG pathology discovery. Reflexive learning models send discovery results back to the psychological motor. It settles on ultimate choices about the patient's state. It appropriately educates the concerned partners about the outcomes. Medical services professionals break down the wellbeing records and results and afterward back to patients.

Proposed Work

The previous work is a medical services framework (Islam, Rahaman, and Islam 2020). It can screen a patient's essential health signal as the room condition. The wired sensors gather information from the patient's body. It employs an ESP32 module and ships off the entryway worker. For the web UI, ThingSpeak aid in for the graphical translation, and show of gathered outcomes. ThingSpeak shows the current status and cycle of exchanges. The HTTP convention gives a simple network to the correspondence between a Wi-Fi module and the webserver. Five sensors catch the information from the clinic climate sensors. They include a heartbeat sensor, internal heat level sensor, room-temperature sensor, CO sensor, and CO2 sensor. The mistake level is inside a specific breaking point for each case. The state of the patients is at the entrance to clinical staff. It can measure and examine the current circumstance of the patients. Table 1 jolts the notations used in the proposal.

Table 1. Notation used in the proposal

Notations used	**Description**
Network considered	N
Identification of the patient	P_{id}
Identification of the doctor	D_{id}
Biometric of the doctor	D_{bio}
Biometric of the patient	P_{bio}
Data	D_i
Server/cloud	S_i
Transmitted time	$Time_i$

Storing Data Using Blockchain

Blockchain (Bai et al. 2019) is a method used in the digital world. It helps to increase reliability in the transactions. In this proposal, the methodology provides authorization to the data stored. The data in the database consists of biometric and identification readings of the doctor and patient (N. Ambika 2020). The hash code is generated using the same.

The database is accessed in the following ways –

- The credentials of the doctor and patient are required. Once the database is created, it does not hinder modifying the created record. It leaves traces of its modification. The procedure starts with registering the credentials of the doctor and the sick. In equation (1), the hash value $Hash_i$ is generated by the server/cloud Si using the credentials of the doctor identification Did, doctor biometric D_{bio}, patient's identification Pid and patient biometric P_{bio}.

$$S_i: Hash_i \leftarrow D_{id}||D_{bio}||P_{id}||P_{bio} \tag{1}$$

- After registration, the data is fed into the account of the patient. The data can vary with the disease diagnosed. In this work, heartbeat, temperature, pulse rate are considered. In equation (2), the data D_i is the assembly of heartbeat H_i, temperature T_i and pulse rate P_i.

$$D_i \rightarrow H_i||T_i||P_i \tag{2}$$

- This data is transmitted to the server, where the hash value of the data sent is prepared. The data is encrypted and stored. In equation (3), the data D_i and time of transmission $Time_i$ is concatenated, and the hash value $Hash_{data}$ is generated by the server S_i.

$$S_i: Hash_{data} \leftarrow D_i||Time_i \tag{3}$$

- The patient or the doctor can access the data as read-only. The patient's or only the doctor's keys make the data to be only read. The credentials of either of them authenticate them and allow them to access the data. Table 2 details the algorithm used to generate the hash code. Table 3 describes the steps used to create the database.

Table 2. Algorithm to generate hash code (registration procedure)

Step 1: Input doctor identification (24 bits), patient identification (24 bits), doctor biometric (40 bits), patient biometric (40 bits)
Step 2: concatenate all the bits
Step 3: Apply right circular shift to 2 positions
Step 4: divide into two halves (64 bits each)
Step 5: Consider the mask bits as 1's (64 1's)
Step 5.1 : Add the first halves bits to the mask bits (64 bits are obtained neglecting the last carry bit)
Step 5.2 : Subtract the second halves bits from the mask bits (64 bits are obtained)
Step 6: Xor the first and second halves bits from left most end (64 bits are obtained)
Step 7: Go to Step 3 if the number of bits > 16 bits
Step 8: Resultant is 16 bits of hash code

Table 3. Steps followed to generate the database

Step 1: The registration process starts by accepting the identities and biometric values of the patient and the doctor.
Step 2: The same is used every time to insert the data. A hash is created (implementing blockchain technique) using the data fed (like heart beat, pulse rate) and time data is fed.
Step 3: If the data is modified, the hash previously generated reveals it.

Simulation and Evaluation of the Work

The proposal is the continuation of the previous work (Islam, Rahaman, and Islam 2020). The suggestion is a medical services framework (Islam, Rahaman, and Islam 2020). It can screen a patient's essential health signal as the room condition. The wired sensors gather information from the patient's body. It employs an ESP32 module and ships off the entryway worker. For the web UI, ThingSpeak aid in for the graphical translation, and show of gathered outcomes. ThingSpeak shows the current status and cycle of exchanges. The HTTP convention gives a simple network to the correspondence between a Wi-Fi module and the webserver. Five sensors catch the information from the clinic climate sensors. They include a heartbeat sensor, internal heat level sensor, room-temperature sensor, CO sensor, and CO_2 sensor. The mistake level is inside a specific breaking point for each case. The state of the patients is at the entrance to clinical staff. It can measure and examine the current circumstance of the patients.

Table 4. Simulation parameters

Parameters used in the proposal	Description
Dimension considered	200m * 200m
Number of devices considered	20
Length of doctor/patient identification	24 bits
Length biometric considered	40 bits
Length of the hash value generated(registration process)	16 bits
Length of data	450 bits
Length of hash value generated (data)	20 bits
Simulation time	50 ms

The suggestion stores the data and provides a management method where only legitimate users can see the records. The procedure commences with the registration stage, where the doctor and the patient credentials are collected. The hash content is generated using credentials. This substance acts as an authenticator in different values. The doctor or the patient can access the details fed earlier using their credentials. To modify and update details, the details of doctor and sick are essential. The data stored after authentication also generates a hash value to adapt reliability in the system. The detection of modification to the storage happens at an earlier stage to take an appropriate decision.

The work is simulated in C++. Table 4 details the parameters used in the work.

Availability of Data

Authentication is a methodology where the communicating party is analyzed for their legitimacy. The first part of the care cloud (Shakil et al. 2020) is chargeable for the management of patients report and alternative data. It has three layers, particularly shopper level, health service supplier level, and information center level. The supplier level divides into body and security levels. The biometric identification agent acts at the protection level. The shopper level provides an associate degree interaction interface between the cloud information and its users. The protection and resource provisioning is successively handled by the two parts of the health service supplier level severally. The storage and its management area unit is the responsibility of the info center level. The Health Information Management System is chargeable for the management, storage, and retrieval of the information. The workers and patients register within the healthcare center area unit. They give their signature samples victimization either the signature capturing device or their smartphones that area unit put in with the signature capturing package. The system captures the user's signature. The standard of the given signature checks victimization SigQuality checker package. The performance of this package confirms the recorded signature samples. It matches up to the standard standards needed for authentication. The options of the samples area unit extracted and area unit keep within the care cloud. The practitioner will be able to view the data after the update. The suggestion enables modification and updating of data. It also allows viewing the data with only the user credentials.

The biometry (N. Ambika 2020) of the personnel and patient extraction generates the individual hash value. It is on the server. Whenever the worker examines the patient, the worker demonstrates himself by giving the biometry and location details. The hash value for identical is generated and cross-verified with the information hold on the server. On positive confirmation, the personnel area unit was allowed to update the analysis outline of the patient. The identical is updated. This value is concatenated with the information and submitted to the server.

Comparing this work to the suggestion location information is necessary. The proposal aims to view the records after authenticating with either of their credentials. The user (doctor/patient) will be able to view the data related to them. To modify or update them, both the credentials become necessary. Comparing to the previous works (N. Ambika 2020 (Shakil et al. 2020), the suggestion increases availability by 33.55%. Figure 1 represents the same.

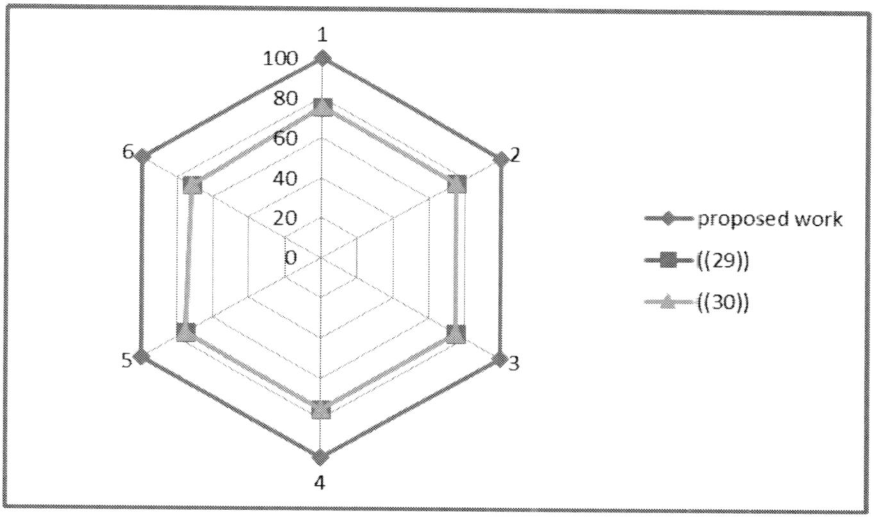

Figure 1. Comparison of availability of data w.r.t previous work.

CONCLUSION

IoT is the smart device used in many applications to gather environmental data. These devices also help in analyzing the data. Health devices and healthcare services deploy these nodes to record patient readings and monitor them. The previous work proposes a medical services framework in an IoT network. It can screen a patient's essential health signal as the room condition. The wired sensors gather information from the patient's body. It employs an ESP32 module and ships off the entryway worker. Five sensors catch the information from the clinic climate sensors. They include a heartbeat sensor, internal heat level sensor, room-temperature sensor, CO sensor, and CO_2 sensor. The mistake level is inside a specific breaking point for each case. The state of the patients is at the entrance to clinical staff. It can measure and examine the current circumstance of the patients. The proposal stores the measured values. These stored quantities can help doctors suggest future treatment for the patient. The proposal increases availability by 33.55% compared with the previous contribution.

REFERENCES

Alhussein, M., G. Muhammad, M. S. Hossain, and S. U. Amin. "Cognitive IoT-cloud integration for smart healthcare: case study for epileptic seizure detection and monitoring." *Mobile Networks and Applications* 23, no. 6 (2018): 1624-1635.

Ambika, N. "Reliable Data Transmission Using Biometric Authentication Methodology in IoT." In *Security and Privacy in the Internet of Things*, by Syed Rameem Zahra and Mohammad Ahsan chishti, 67-78. CRC PRESS, 2020.

Ambika, N. "Methodical IoT-Based Information System in Healthcare." In *Smart Medical Data Sensing and IoT Systems Design in Healthcare*, by Chinmay Chakraborty (eds.), 155-177. US: IGI Global., 2020.

Amin, S. U., M. S. Hossain, G. Muhammad, M. Alhussein, and M. A. Rahman. "Cognitive smart healthcare for pathology detection and monitoring." *IEEE Access* 7 (2019): 10745-10753.

Bai, L., M. Hu, M. Liu, and J. Wang. "BPIIoT: A light-weighted blockchain-based platform for Industrial IoT." *IEEE Access* 7 (2019): 58381-58393.

Banka, S., I. Madan, and S. S. Saranya. "Smart healthcare monitoring using IoT." *International Journal of Applied Engineering Research* 13, no. 15 (2018): 11984-11989.

Bansal, M., and B. Gandhi. "IoT based development boards for Smart Healthcare Applications." *4th International Conference on Computing Communication and Automation (ICCCA).* Greater Noida, India: IEEE, 2018. 1-7.

BK, B., and K. N. Muralidhara. "Secured smart healthcare monitoring system based on Iot." *International Journal on Recent and Innovation Trends in Computing and Communication* 3, no. 7 (2015): 4958-4961.

Budida, D. A. M., and R. S. Mangrulkar. "Design and implementation of smart HealthCare system using IoT." *International Conference on Innovations in Information, Embedded and Communication Systems (ICIIECS)* . Coimbatore, India: IEEE., 2017. 1-7.

Catarinucci, L., et al. "An IoT-aware architecture for smart healthcare systems." *IEEE internet of things journal* 2, no. 6 (2015): 515-526.

Dautov, R., S. Distefano, and R. Buyya. "Hierarchical data fusion for Smart Healthcare." *Journal of Big Data* 6, no. 1 (2019): 1-23.

Gong, T., H. Huang, P. Li, K. Zhang, and H. Jiang. "A medical healthcare system for privacy protection based on IoT." *Seventh International Symposium on Parallel Architectures, Algorithms and Programming (PAAP).* Nanjing, China: IEEE, 2015. 217-222.

Gupta, P., D. Agrawal, J. Chhabra, and P. K. Dhir. "IoT based smart healthcare kit." *International Conference on Computational Techniques in Information and Communication Technologies (ICCTICT).* New Delhi, India: IEEE., 2016. 237-242.

Hussain, T., K. Muhammad, S. Khan, A. Ullah, M. Y. Lee, and S. W. Baik. "Intelligent baby behavior monitoring using embedded vision in IoT for smart healthcare centers." *Journal of Artificial Intelligence and Systems* 1, no. 1 (2019): 110-124.

Islam, M. M., A. Rahaman, and M. R. Islam. "Development of smart healthcare monitoring system in IoT environment." *SN computer science* 1 (2020): 1-11.

Jeong, J. S., O. Han, and Y. Y. You. "A design characteristics of smart healthcare system as the IoT application." *Indian Journal of Science and Technology* 9, no. 37 (2016): 1-8.

Jia, X., Q. Feng, T. Fan, and Q. Lei. "RFID technology and its applications in Internet of Things (IoT)." *2nd international conference on consumer electronics, communications and networks (CECNet).* Yichang, China: IEEE, 2012. 1282-1285.

Khan, J., et al. "SMSH: secure surveillance mechanism on smart healthcare IoT system with probabilistic image encryption." *IEEE Access* 8 (2020): 15747-15767.

Mehdi Khosrow-Pour, D. B. A., (Eds.). *Encyclopedia of Information Science and Technology, Fifth Edition.* USA: IGI Publications, 2020.

Mohapatra, S., S. Mohanty, and S. Mohanty. "Smart healthcare: an approach for ubiquitous healthcare management using IoT." *Big Data Analytics for Intelligent Healthcare Management*, 2019: 175-196.

Nagaraj, A. *Introduction to Sensors in IoT and Cloud Computing Applications.* UAE: Bentham Science Publishers, 2021.

Naik, S., and E Sudarshan. "Smart healthcare monitoring system using raspberry Pi on IoT platform." *ARPN Journal of Engineering and Applied Sciences* 14, no. 4 (2019): 872-876.

Patan, R., G. P. Ghantasala, R. Sekaran, D. Gupta, and M. Ramachandran. "Smart healthcare and quality of service in IoT using grey filter convolutional based cyber physical system." *Sustainable Cities and Society*, 2020: 1-54.

Salahuddin, M. A., A. Al-Fuqaha, M. Guizani, K. Shuaib, and F. Sallabi. "Softwarization of internet of things infrastructure for secure and smart healthcare." *Computers and Society*, May 28, 2018: 1-9.

Shakil, K. A., F. J. Zareen, M. Alam, and S. Jabin. "BAMHealthCloud: A biometric authentication and data management system for healthcare data in cloud." *Journal of King Saud University-Computer and Information Sciences* 32, no. 1 (January 2020): 57-64.

Tuli, S., et al. "HealthFog: An ensemble deep learning based Smart Healthcare System for Automatic Diagnosis of Heart Diseases in integrated IoT and fog computing environments." *Future Generation Computer Systems* 104 (2020): 187-200.

Ullah, A., I. Sehr, M. Akbar, and H. Ning. "FoG assisted secure de-duplicated data dissemination in smart healthcare IoT." *IEEE International Conference on Smart Internet of Things (SmartIoT).* Xi'an, China: IEEE., 2018 . 166-171.

Whitmore, A., A. Agarwal, and L. Da Xu. "The Internet of Things—A survey of topics and trends." *Information Systems Frontiers* 17, no. 2 (2015): 261-274.

Yang, Z., Q. Zhou, L. Lei, K. Zheng, and W. Xiang. "An IoT-cloud based wearable ECG monitoring system for smart healthcare." *Journal of medical systems* 40, no. 12 (2016): 1-11.

Zhu, H., et al. "Smart healthcare in the era of internet-of-things." *IEEE Consumer Electronics Magazine* 8, no. 5 (2019): 26-30.

About the Editors

Parma Nand is PhD. in Computer Science & Engineering from IIT Roorkee, M.Tech & B.Tech in Computer Science & Engineering from IIT Delhi. Prof Parma Nand has more than 27 years of experience both in industry and academia. He has received various awards like best teacher award from Union Minister, best students project guide award from Microsoft in 2015 and best faculty award from cognizant in 2016. He had successfully completed government funded projects and spearheaded the last five IEEE International conferences on Computing, Communication & Automation (ICCCA), IEEE students chapters, Technovation Hackathon 2019, Technovation Hackathon 2020, International Conference on Computing, Communication, and Intelligent Systems (ICCCIS-2021). He is a member of the Executive Council of IEEE UP section (R-10), the Executive Committee IEEE Computer and Signal Processing Society, the India council Computer Society, the Executive Council Computer Society of India, Noida section and has acted as an observer in many IEEE conferences. He also has active memberships of ACM, IEEE, CSI, ACEEE, ISOC, IAENG, and IASCIT. He is a lifetime member of the Soft Computing Research Society (SCRS) and ISTE. He has delivered many talks at International & National Conferences/ Workshops/Seminars in India & abroad. He has published more than 150 papers in peer reviewed international/national journals and conferences.

He has also published a number of book chapters in reputed publications like Springer Berlin Heidelberg. He has reviewed a number of books for publications like Tata McGraw-Hill, Galgotias Publications etc. and papers in journals of international repute. He is an active member of advisory/technical program committee of reputed International/National conferences & reviewer of number of reputed Journals, e.g., Springer, Elsevier Journal Computers & Electrical Engineering. His research interest includes Computer Graphics, Algorithm, Distributed Computing and Wireless and Sensor networking.

Arun Prakash Agrawal is currently working as a Professor with Department of Computer Science and Engineering at Sharda University, Greater Noida, India. He obtained his PhD and Master's in Computer Science and Engineering from Guru Gobind Singh Indraprastha University, New Delhi, India. He was the gold medalist of his batch. Prior to his current assignment, he served in many academic institutions including Amity University, Noida. He has several research papers to his credit in refereed journals and conferences of international repute in India and abroad, including Journal of Neural Computing and Applications published by Springer. He has also taught short-term courses at Swinburne University of Technology, Melbourne, Australia and Amity Global Business School, Singapore. His research interests include Machine Learning, Software Testing, Artificial Intelligence and Soft Computing.

Ankur Choudhary majored in computer science and engineering and pursued a PhD from the School of ICT, Gautam Buddha University (GBU), Greater Noida, India. He has approximately 15+ years of teaching experience and is currently a professor at Sharda Univeristy, Greater Noida, India. His areas of research include: nature-inspired optimization, artificial intelligence, software engineering, medical image processing, and digital watermarking. Dr. Choudhary has published research papers in various SCI/Scopus indexed international conferences and journals, and is associated with various international journals as a reviewer and editorial board member. He has organized conferences, special sessions at international conferences, and served and delivered as session chair.

Vishal Jain is an Associate Professor in the Department of Computer Science and Engineering, School of Engineering and Technology, Sharda University, Greater Noida, U. P., India. Before that, he worked for several years as an Associate Professor at Bharati Vidyapeeth's Institute of Computer Applications and Management (BVICAM), New Delhi. He has more than 14 years of experience in academics. He has more than 480 research citation indices with Google Scholar (h-index score 12 and i-10 index 16). He has authored more than 85 research papers in reputed conferences and journals, including the Web of Science and Scopus. He has authored and edited more than 15 books with various reputed publishers, including Elsevier, Springer, DeGruyter, Apple Academic Press, CRC, Taylor and Francis Group, Scrivener, Wiley, Emerald, and IGI-Global. His research areas include information retrieval, semantic web, ontology engineering, data mining, ad hoc networks, and sensor networks. He received a Young Active Member Award for the year 2012–13 from the Computer Society of India and a Best Faculty Award for the year 2017 and Best Researcher Award for the year 2019 from BVICAM, New Delhi. He holds PhD (CSE), M.Tech (CSE), MBA (HR), MCA, MCP and CCNA.

INDEX

A

B

C

D

E

F

G

H

I

L

M

N

O

P

Q

R

S

T

U

V

W

Y